# Pseudogout

## Living With Pseudogout

A guide to understanding, coping with, and treating Pseudogout, including exercise tips.

by

Howard Heverdon

D1211938

## Disclaimer

# Table of Contents

# Introduction

Arthritis is a disease that can progressively become very serious and is tremendously debilitating in its nature. It is often believed that this disease can only affect seniors; however, arthritis can be found in people regardless of their age. There are over a 100 different types of arthritis currently known to medical science. With so many types of arthritis out there, one key component of the treatment is to first identify the type of arthritis present. Even though there are many types of arthritis, they commonly share the same types of symptoms. For example, one of the most common symptoms that are present in almost every kind of arthritis is joint pain. This joint paint can be extreme in the morning, and may go away in an hour or so, only to come back at night at its peak.

It is not unusual for physical movements to make the joint pain even worse; this is something that is the result of little fragments of bone breaking off. For many people, the pain gets worse if they remain idle for an extended period of time, such as when watching television or sitting. Being seated in a car for too long is also known to cause pain in the joints. If a person tends to stay still in order to avoid pain, they simply end up in a cycle where they experience intense pain when they eventually move.

Even though joint pain is the most common symptom of arthritis, there are many other ways in which arthritis affects the body. For example, there are certain types of arthritis that affect other organs in the body and can cause a physical deformity. Some arthritis cause scaly blemishes on the skin while also affecting people's moods and causing them to feel tired, worried and uneasy.

This book will focus on a particular type of arthritis rather than providing a generic overview of the disease. The kind of arthritis this book will focus on is called *Pseudogout*, a type of acute arthritis that is caused by calcium pyrophosphate crystals.

# Chapter 1: Understanding Pseudogout

## What is Pseudogout?

Arthritis is a family of complex musculoskeletal diseases that comprise of over a hundred different conditions that destroy bones, joints, cartilage, muscles, and other tissues, thereby halting or hampering physical movements.

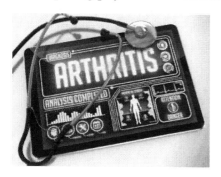

Pseudogout is one of the conditions that belong to the arthritis family, and is a result of *calcium pyrophosphate dehydrate (CPPD) crystal deposition disease.* CPPD is a crystal deposition disease that results when crystals accumulate in the joints and in the tissues that surround the joints. These deposits of calcium induce inflammation in the joints and can break down the cartilage found inside the joint.

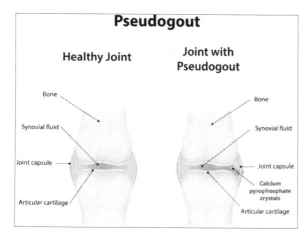

Out of all CPPD cases, 25 percent are those of pseudogout.

## Effects

Calcium pyrophosphate dehydrate (CPPD) disease can cause crystals to build up in the joints in a number of ways.

Here are the effects of calcium pyrophosphate dehydrate (CPPD) crystal deposition disease:

- Sudden inception of intense, consistent pain in a single joint; the joint may be red, hot, stiff and swollen. In general, the average attack is less intense than in gout.
- A single attack can last from a few days to around two weeks.
- Almost half of all attacks are centered on the knee (compared to gout's fondness for the big toe).
- The acute attack may be accompanied by a fever.
- The time between attacks is usually completely painless.
- Attacks can occur suddenly, or may or be induced by surgery, trauma, or severe illness (such as heart attack or stroke).
- After the attacks, damage to the join progresses for years. The cartilage found inside the joints may break and the pieces floating between the joints will induce additional pain. As the cartilage erodes away, the bones rub together and cause a stiffening of the joints.

## Symptoms

Many kinds of arthritis occur slowly and gradually over a certain period of time. In its early stages, an individual may experience mild pain occasionally. In comparison, pseudogout strikes suddenly and without any warning. It can cause severe pain, leading the affected person to believe that it is a life-threatening situation; as a matter of fact, it is not rare for an accurate diagnosis to be prolonged just because more serious conditions are being considered.

The usual symptoms of pseudogout are as follows:

### A greater joint area is involved

Pseudogout affects the knee, elbow, shoulder, wrist, ankle, large knuckles, spine or hip. This is a much larger area compared to that affected by gout (another form of arthritis), which includes the fingertips, heel, big toe and instep.

### Pain

One of the most noticeable symptoms includes excruciating pain at the joints affected by pseudogout.

### Swelling

Fluid build-up in the affected joints can lead to extensive swelling.

### Discoloration

The skin around the join may turn purple or red.

### Warmth

The skin will be warm to the touch around the affected areas.

### Stiffness

The combined effect of pain and swelling may reduce the range of motion of the joints and make them stiff.

### Rapid Onset

Pseudogout can develop quickly and without any signs at all. It takes around 6 to 12 hours for the swelling and the pain to reach its peak.

### Short Duration

If left untreated, a pseudogout attack can last for 5 to 14 days. The pain fades away with time. No symptoms are present in between the attacks or episodes.

### Fever

Due to the fact that the immune system reacts to the crystals of calcium pyrophosphate, a fever may develop.

## Causes

A lot needs to be found concerning the reasons behind the build-up of calcium pyrophosphate crystals in the joints, including studying the role of these crystals in causing a pseudogout attack. The known causes and risk factors of pseudogout are as follows:

### *Age*

The majority of people who develop this disease are aged 60 or above. The chances of developing pseudogout increases with age, and according to the American College of Rheumatology, the presence of calcium pyrophosphate crystals increase by a mere 3 per cent when people are in their 60s. By the time a person reaches his or her 90s, the increase in crystals is as high as 50 per cent.

### *Joint Trauma*

A surgery, trauma, or sepsis can cause a pseudogout flare up. According to experts, a trauma can cause the cartilage in a joint to shed calcium phosphate crystals that have been collected inside it. Once they have been shed, the crystals can trigger the immune system, which is the primary cause behind the swelling and numerous other symptoms of this disease.

### *Family History*

Genetics play a strong role and make some people prone to calcium pyrophosphate crystals within their joints. According to the latest research, a particular mutation found in the ANKH gene can make people more likely to develop pseudogout, and that too at an early age compared to those people who do not have the genetic mutation.

## Diagnosis

You may have banged your elbow on the doorframe and now the pain and swelling seems to have increased tremendously; the reason behind this may be that your apparently innocent trauma might have triggered a flare-up of pseudogout – a crystal-induced arthritis. Whenever you experience extreme pain and can see swelling, such as in the situation mentioned above, it is advisable that you go and see a doctor.

### Diagnosing Pseudogout
Pseudogout and gout are both a result of the deposition of large crystals in the joints; however, they are caused by different types of crystals. Pseudogout is a result of calcium pyrophosphate dehydrate (CPPD) crystals, whereas gout is causes by crystals of sodium urate.

One of the major challenges involved in correctly diagnosing pseudogout is distinguishing it from other forms of arthritis and rheumatic diseases. Besides resembling the symptoms of gout, the symptoms of pseudogout can closely resemble those of:

- Rheumatoid arthritis
- Infectious arthritis
- Osteoarthritis
- Ankylosing spondylitis

Nonetheless, the symptoms that you describe to your doctor will be of a particular help in making sure that the doctor makes a correct diagnosis. For instance, gout typically starts in the big toe, whereas pseudogout is known to develop in the knee.

The following information reveals the general process that doctors use to diagnose pseudogout and differentiate it from other types of arthritis.

### Health History
Doctors, when diagnosing pseudogout, start off by asking questions about the health history of the concerned individual. They ask about any medical conditions that may already be present in order to determine whether something has triggered the symptoms or not, for example, some infection or a trauma to the inflamed joint.

According to Kevin Deane, MD, who is an assistant professor of medicine at the University of Colorado Health Sciences Center's rheumatology division, says:

*"Pseudogout can be associated with other diseases that need to be investigated. With pseudogout you usually try and identify if there is a long-term disease that might be driving it. If that's not driving it, you basically have to put them on long term anti-inflammatory medications."*

### Examinations
The next thing in the process of diagnosing pseudogout is a physical examination where the joint or joints are checked by the doctor to see how well they can be moved.

If the doctor suspects the presence of pseudogout, he or she extracts some fluid from the affected joint. When this fluid is observed under a polarizing microscope, the crystals – if they are present in the fluid – can be seen. Brick-shaped crystals imply that pseudogout is present, whereas needle-shaped ones are indicative of gout.

The fluid may also be cultured to determine whether there is an infection in the joint or not. According to a clinical professor at Tulane University of Medicine in New Orleans, both pseudogout and joint infection can be present at the same time.

An X-ray can also reveal a build-up of calcium deposits in the joints. However, the x-ray will not be able to tell the doctor specifically that you have pseudogout. A lot of people have calcium crystals in their joints, but they never develop symptoms of pseudogout or if they do, it is only after a traumatic injury to the joint.

### The Aftermath
Once pseudogout has been confirmed, the healthcare professional will make a treatment plan for your condition.

Unlike gout, where patients can take medicine to bring down the uric acid level that causes it, there is no medicine that can remove calcium deposits from the affected joint. Corticosteroids and anti-inflammatory medicines are prescribed to treat a flare up. There are also some medications that can prevent a flare up in people that are prone to them.

## Treatment

As mentioned in the previous sub-section, there is no treatment available that can remove the calcium pyrophosphate crystals from the joint once they have been deposited. Whenever pseudogout has been caused by a known condition, such as hyperthyroidism, then measures are taken to treat the primary illness, which in turn tends to diminish or reduce pseudogout episodes. On the other hand, pseudogout is frequently *idiopathic* – meaning that it has no obvious cause – the treatment in this case only focuses on relieving the symptoms rather than preventing them.

If a person takes measures to control the inflammation in the joint, along with controlling other symptoms, the amount of damage that occurs to the joint in each pseudogout episode can be limited.

The steps to ease the symptoms of pseudogout typically include the following:

**Ice** – A cool compress can be applied to the affected joint or joints in an attempt to reduce discomfort and decrease the amount of swelling.

**Rest** – It can be very painful to use the joint that has been affected by pseudogout. It is recommended that those individuals who have this condition rest the affected joint in order to alleviate pain and swelling.

**Elevation** – Whenever possible, the affected limb should be elevated to reduce swelling. For instance, if the knee joint is affected by pseudogout, the knee should be slightly more elevated than the body when either sitting down or lying.

## Other Methods to Alleviate Symptoms

The following methods are often used to help a person deal with the symptoms of pseudogout.

**Aspiration** – A doctor can aspirate the affected joint by inserting a needle into it and removing the synovial fluid, which would have accumulated in the joint. This process relieves the stress in the joint and provides added comfort to the affected person. This treatment method is often used in conjunction with steroid injections.

**Corticosteroids Injections** – Corticosteroids may be injected into the inflamed joint in order to relieve pain. This method is popular among those people who have sensitivities to certain medicines.

**Oral Steroids** – If two or more joints are affected by pseudogout, then corticosteroid injections are considered to be impractical. In this case, oral steroids may be recommended. For those people who cannot tolerate colchicine, or NSAIDs, oral steroids can be very useful.

# Chapter 2: Natural & Alternative Remedies

There are numerous natural and alternative remedies available that have been known to bring relief to people with arthritic conditions, including pseudogout. While it is true that there is no cure available for musculoskeletal diseases such as pseudogout and gout, these remedies can help to prevent the condition from worsening and alleviate the pain associated with such diseases.

This chapter will highlight some things that will have a positive effect in helping you manage your medical condition. All the remedies depicted below have scientific backing and have been proven to have constructive results.

## Disinfecting Your Mouth Regularly

Brushing your teeth regularly has more benefits than just keeping your teeth and gums clean and healthy. A growing number of researchers have confirmed that the type of bacteria that infects our gums may also be the cause of certain types of arthritis. In one study, the bacteria that cause many cases of gingivitis infections were also found many arthritis patients' joint synovial fluid.

The ideal way to go about preventing these bacteria from causing or aggravating your arthritic condition (including pseudogout) is to disinfect your mouth regularly by brushing your teeth and by rinsing your mouth with a disinfectant mouthwash.

### How to Do This:

You do not have to use chemicals to clean your mouth. In fact, you can use certain things right out of your kitchen, such as baking soda. Add 1 tablespoon of baking soda to a cup of water and rinse your mouth. This can be followed by rinsing with the mixture of a few drops of food-grade Lavender essential oil and

Rosemary essential oil in a cup of water. Make sure you do not swallow the essential oils.

## Turmeric

The main polyphenol in turmeric is known as curcumin and it has been proven to have several hundred health benefits, with one of them being its powerful anti-inflammation and anti-pain abilities.

According to studies, turmeric is a powerful herb that is highly effective in combating pain and inflammation associated with pseudogout and other arthritis conditions.

Curcumin is extremely safe to use. A safety study carried out in 2010 found that doses as high as 8 grams each day are perfectly tolerated by the body. However, just like any herb, it is important to take care when consuming it along with any other synthetic medication. Consult your doctor to be on the safe side.

**How to Use It:**

<u>Cooking</u> – Turmeric can be added to foods during preparation. It is recommended that you consume turmeric with healthy fat such as olive oil. In addition, you may want to add turmeric to rice, eggs, soups, pasta, and sauces. The possibilities are actually endless.

<u>Green Juice</u> – Add between a half and one tablespoon of turmeric to your green juice.

<u>Supplements</u> – There are various turmeric supplements out there and you may want to ask your physician for a recommendation.

## Infrared Light Therapy

There is no doubt that infrared light therapy is among one of the best ways to relieve joint pain. Even though its advantages have been scientifically proven, very few people are aware of this effective, drug-free method of relieving pain.

During the last 40 years, studies have found some remarkably powerful therapeutic benefits of light for the human body. Both infrared and visible red light have shown at least around 24 numerous types of changes at cellular levels. There is solid evidence that tells us that infrared can soothe inflammation and reduce pain efficiently.

Infrared therapy is already used to relieve pain associated with Lyme and Fibromyalgia diseases. It can also be used for arthritis-like diseases such as pseudogout to reduce the inflammation and pain.

Infrared light at 880nm is able to penetrate to a depth of around 30 to 40 mm, making it highly effective for joint pain, bone pain, and deep muscle issues. Even though no heat is involved, it can heal inflammation.

Infrared rays are completely safe, and they must not be confused with ultraviolet rays that are known to cause, in excessive amounts, sun burn and skin cancer. As a matter of fact, it is so safe that it is commonly used in neonatal care units to keep new-borns warm.

**How to Use It:**

There are numerous ways in which infrared rays can be used at home safely and conveniently. One way is to use an infrared heating mat.

**Infrared Heating Pads** – The best pads usually use natural stones such as Jade. These emit infrared radiation directly onto the inflamed and painful areas. They can induce instant relief that can last for several hours, thereby completely eliminating the need for many pain-killing medications altogether.

**Infrared Sauna Blanket** – Even though these blankets can be quite expensive, these often turn out to be the best infrared option for many.

## Cod Liver Oil

Cod liver oil is a supplement that is extracted from the liver of codfish. This is rich in omega-3 fatty acids, docosahexaenoic acid (DHA) and eicosapentaenoic acid (EPA). It also contains rich quantities of Vitamin A and D.

According to one study, around 2 teaspoons of cod liver oil each day can reduce the number of painkillers required to relieve pain associated with pseudogout.

While another study highlighted the benefits of reduced morning stiffness, pain intensity and swollen joints as a result of consuming a gram of cod liver oil each day.

Just like other supplements, it is advised not to mix cod liver oil with any other medication. Consult your healthcare professional before you make this a part of your daily intake. High doses of cod liver oil can be potentially dangerous.

**How to Use It:**

Take 1 or 2 tablets each day after your meal. Ask your physician for a recommendation.

## Ginger

In terms of documented benefits for joint relief, ginger stands second preceded by turmeric. For instance, one study states that ginger has a number of compounds that have strong effects in relieving pain associated with joint-related issues, such as pseudogout and rheumatoid arthritis.

Ginger is extremely safe to use; particularly when consumed in its natural form. If you prefer to take a supplement, you must consult your doctor first.

**How to Use It:**

Fresh ginger is undoubtedly among one of the tastiest foods. It can enhance the taste of chicken soup, and can also be paired with fruits such as apples and banana as well as meats such as chicken and turkey. Do not forget gingerbread and ginger ale.

*Ginger tea* is also effective in controlling pseudogout flare-ups, and if you feel as if you are developing one, you can slice a few pieces of ginger along with a few pieces of turmeric and boil them together (in water) for ten minutes. Add a touch of lemon and honey to make a tasty pain-relieving tea.

*Herbal mix* consisting of ginger power, cinnamon power and turmeric powder is also quite effective in reducing inflammation and pain. Mix all these together and take 1 tablespoon of this mixture in your green juice or coffee every day.

## Glucosamin-Choindroitin–Quercitin Combo (GCQG)

This is an extremely powerful and effective combo that can be used to reduce inflammation and arthritis-related symptoms. A number of studies have proven that GCQG has a strong pain-relieving effect.

Chondroitin and Glucosamine are types of naturally occurring sugar that are believed to help the body in repairing damaged cartilage in joints and enhance joint movement as well as flexibility.

It is absolutely important that diabetic patients avoid using this supplement at all costs because it can cause their blood sugar levels to spike. In addition, it is recommended that you consult your doctor before taking these supplements.

GCQG is a supplement, and can therefore be only used as such.

## Krill Oil

New emerging information suggests that fatty acids extracted from shrimp-like organisms, such as krill, can be quite effective in decreasing joint inflammation due to their natural anti-inflammatory compounds.

Krill oil contains fatty acids that are quite similar to those found in fish oil. These fats are believed to reduce swelling, make blood platelets less sticky, and bring down cholesterol. When the blood platelets are less sticky, they are less probable to develop clots.

A study carried out by the US National Library of Medicine found that a daily dose of Neptune Krill Oil amounting to 300 mg could have significant effects in reducing the inflammation and pain linked with pseudogout. The treatment period is relatively short, with prominent effects appearing within 7 to 14 days.

When used appropriately for a relatively short period of time (up to three months), krill oil is safe for adults. It is important that you do not use krill oil if you are allergic or sensitive to seafood. It is recommended, like for all supplements, to consult a healthcare professional.

Krill oil can only be used by consuming krill oil supplements.

## Rosehip Powder

Rosehips are the round portion just below the petals of a rose flower. Rosehips contain the seeds of the plant. A recent study found that rosehip is almost three times more effective in relieving pain than paracetamol. In addition, it was found to be 40% more effective than the drug glucosamine.

Rosehips are also a rich source of Vitamin C – a vitamin that increases the body's ability to fight infections and diseases.

It was found during the studies that rosehip has no side effects that are typically associated with pain management drugs, such as drowsiness and constipation. However, it is still important to consult a physician before going for this form of treatment.

### How to Use It:

The best way to gain the benefits of rosehip is to eat it in its powdered form. You can add it to a cup of warm water, or you can even add it to your green juice. If you want a bit more flavour, mix it with ice cream.

## Aromatherapy

Aromatherapy has huge benefits and found to be highly effective in reducing pain and level of depression in pseudogout patients. The study found the following essential oils to be very useful when blended in a proportions of 2:1:2:1:1 -

- Lavender oil
- Marjoram
- Eucalyptus
- Rosemary
- Peppermint

Mix in carrier oil comprising of almond (45 pc), apricot (45 pc), and jojoba oil (10 pc). After blending, they should be diluted to 1.5 per cent.

### How to Use It:

It is a good idea to avoid making your own aromatherapy formulas and settle for well-known brands that are available on the market. These formulas have typically been created to offer maximum effectiveness.

## Eggshell Membrane

The eggshell membrane contains a powerful concoction of effective minerals, proteins and vitamins. It was also, recently, proved to diminish inflammation and pain associated with pseudogout and other forms of arthritis and musculoskeletal degenerative diseases.

The National Osteoporosis Foundation conducted a trial in which they found that 500 mg of eggshell membrane taken over a period of ten days actually reduced joint pain as well as stiffness.

A study related to eggshell membrane was also published in *Clinical Interventions in Aging* journal. This study revealed that people who took a minimum of 500 mg of eggshell membrane for a month reported to be completely free of pain.

## Gelatin

A mega-analysis by the National Institute of Health revealed that ingested gelatin increased the joint cartilage in animals.

The pain and inflammation tend to reduce well before the build-up of cartilage; gelatin tends to have the effect of aspirin or cortisol on the cartilage.

Gelatin is FDA-approved as a dietary supplement for adults.

### How to Use It:

Gelatin can be added to oatmeal and smoothies, along with salads, seafood dishes, and meat. This will increase the value of a meal.

To ensure that you do not lose the nutrients found in gelatin, do not warm it.

## Five Natural Methods Backed by Science for Reducing the Symptoms of Pseudogout

Finding the right kind of home remedies for pseudogout, rheumatoid arthritis, osteoarthritis, and other types of arthritis is fairly easy. However, it is difficult to find effective remedies that actually work. Only a few of these have been thoroughly studied; even those remedies that have shown promising results in trials do not always work well for everyone out there.

Here are 5 low-risk therapies that have proven to have significant effects in pain reduction and the reduction of inflammation:

*Ice Massage* – Just by rubbing ice cubes in a circular motion over the affected areas can not only reduce swelling, but can also slow the pain signals and restrict the production of chemicals that lead to inflammation. The American College of Rheumatology (ACR) recommends that you carry out ice massage for five to ten minutes a few times a day.

*Fish* – Some fish contain omega-3 that is known to halt the production of chemicals that contribute to inflammation. They are also known to reduce pain. Eat sardines, salmon, tuna, and herring several times a week

*Walking* - There are rarely any therapies that can match the benefits of walking. Walking will not only eliminate stiffness, but it will also reduce pain, build muscles, and enhance your flexibility. Start slow, but try to increase the time to 30 minutes each day.

*Green Tea* – Green tea contains a potent antioxidant called epigallocatechin-3-gallate (EGCG). EGCG is known to block the production of molecules that impose damage upon joints, especially in people with arthritis. Drink 2 to 3 cups of green tea every day to enjoy the benefits.

*Probiotics* – Certain types of probiotic bacteria – such as those found in yoghurt – can reduce pain and eliminate disability issues in people with pseudogout, RA, and other forms of arthritis. Eat yoghurt on a daily basis for a period of 3 months and you will surely see positive results.

## Physical Therapy

The inability to perform certain activities is something that causes people to seek help of their healthcare professionals; this reason is more than that of pain or joint stiffness. If your condition is causing any hindrance in your day-to-day activities, you can consult a physical therapist.

Physical therapists are professionals with extensive clinical experience who are capable of examining, diagnosing, and then preventing or treating conditions that limit your body's movement and functioning on a daily basis. The American Physical Therapy Association (APTA) is the body that oversees these professionals.

Doreen Stiskal, an associate professor at the Seton Hall University in New Jersey, says:

*"The best way to talk about this health profession is that we are movement specialists. When you think about movement, that can be anything from getting in and out of chairs to climbing stairs, to walking in your environment to playing a sport or doing recreational activities."*

*"Physical therapy focuses on the body's ability to do movement."* she adds.

Physical therapy usually consists of several methods and techniques, including the use of splints and braces to support joints, while shoe inserts are used to reduce stress on the lower extremities, as well as cold and hot therapy to alleviate joint stiffness and pain. It also includes several changes to your environment. This includes introducing ergonomic chairs, desks and even chef's mats inside your kitchen. But for the majority of people the main focus of physical therapy is on developing a plan that consists of numerous exercises to enhance their strength, flexibility, balance, and coordination. Stiskal says:

*"All of these, when you put them together, translate into optimal physical function."*

## Directed Therapy

If you have had physical therapy previously and want to pursue it yet again, you may notice something different this time. For example, in the past, your physical therapist might have carried out extensive hot & cold therapy or may have spent a lot of time in going through certain exercises. However, with changes to the healthcare and insurance systems, the time of each of the visits, the number of visits to a physical therapist as well as the entire approach taken by physical therapists has changed. It has now become more productive for your physical therapist to actually spend time teaching you how do all of these things by yourself.

*"We often have short, focused visits. The major goals of physical therapy now are to look at the problems with physical function and give strategies for care."* says Stiskal.

The key to a successful outcome is to learn exercises from your physical therapist and then practice them on your own at home. The body can only get sturdy and powerful with time, provided that continuous efforts are put in to accomplish this. This requires a person to consistently practice the exercises that he or she has been taught by a physical therapist.

The best thing about this new approach is the fact that that it enables a person to have greater control and an important role to play in self-care for long-lasting results. If you have been experiencing a change, such as flare-ups in your pseudogout, which are causing you to lag behind in the exercise program or if there is an of involvement another, different joint which is affecting another area's function, then you may want to return to a physical therapist to get your exercise regime and treatment strategy updated.

Stiskal adds:

*"You can think of physical therapy very much like seeing your physician. You don't need to go to your physician every week to manage your arthritis. Just as you see your physician periodically, you periodically might want to revisit your PT to get an update on your program."*

### *Seeing a Physical Therapist (PT)*
Most of the states in the US provide direct access to a PT. This means that in order to see a physical therapist, you do not need to have a referral from a doctor. However, your insurance company may need doctor's referral if you want them to cover your physical therapy. Your insurance provider will properly also limit the number of sessions for a certain type of problem.

When you do visit a therapist, make sure you think about what your actual problem is. Think about what you want to achieve: do you want to be able to walk around without any pain whatsoever? Do you want to be able to bend your knees and experience no pain? All of this will help you work out a proper therapy plan with your physical therapist – a plan that can effectively reduce your pseudogout-related pain.

## Occupational Therapy

Having arthritis can make even the simplest of everyday tasks painful and difficult. In some cases, using a knife or even turning a key can be quite challenging.

Occupational therapy can make these difficult tasks much easier for you, provided that you work with a therapist who assists people with the pseudogout condition. These types of occupational therapists can help people with arthritis to live life to the fullest by enhancing their capacity to partake in activities, enhancing their quality of life and promoting safety. You can benefit more by getting in touch with an occupational therapist as soon as possible.

The best time to see an occupational therapist is right after you have been diagnosed with pseudogout or other types of arthritis. Your healthcare provider can refer you to an occupational therapist that will enable you to learn about how you can engage in the maximum number of activities with maximum convenience.

An occupational therapist at a renowned therapy centre in NY State explains:

*"We want to know how they're doing with any daily activities such as school, homemaking, work, things like laundry or anything that might become challenging, no matter how large or small. Then we come up with an appropriate plan to address all those issues. My goal is to teach them self-management skills as much as possible."*

This plan can include custom-fitting supports or splints, which can relieve the stress from your joints, eliminate pain, and help avert deformity. Occupational therapists also instruct people on how they can protect their joints by performing activities in a slightly different manner; for instance, using an assistive device or utilizing both hands to do a job.

*"People with arthritis really benefit from assistive devices because they help them do more tasks with less pain,"* says Dodge, an occupational therapist, *"I also focus a lot on home exercise programs that will help increase their range of motion, flexibility, and strength. My goal is to improve their strength so that they can do certain functional activities like turning doorknobs, and then encourage them to continue an exercise plan on their own at home after they've reached a certain strength level."*

It isn't a problem if you choose not to work with an occupational therapist right after being diagnosed with arthritis. If you ever feel the need to seek occupational therapy later in your life, you can choose to do so at any point in time. A lot of people with pseudogout prefer to seek occupational therapy as soon as they realise that their medical condition is making things difficult for them in their day-to-day life. For example, they may start experiencing problems when buttoning a shirt and other simple activities.

Regarding this, Carole Dodge, who is an occupational therapist as well as an Allied Health Supervisor & Clinical Specialist at University of Michigan Hospital's Physical Medicine and Rehabilitation Occupational Therapy Division, says:

*"Arthritis is a chronic disease, so it will continue and change over time. Occupational therapy is always a good option for learning how to overcome some of life's challenges when you have arthritis."*

## Utilizing Heat and Cold for Relieving Pain
Two of the least expensive, simplest, and highly effective methods of reducing pain are heat and cold treatments.

Heat treatments, especially warm baths and the use of heat pads, work surprisingly well for soothing tired muscles and stiff joints.

Heat is particularly great for allowing your body to limber and for getting it ready for a particular physical activity, such as exercise. Cold treatments, on the other hand, are ideal for acute pain, decreasing swelling, decreasing inflammation, and for numbing painful areas.

There are numerous types of heat and cold therapy available. Try out some of the ideas given below and see which ones offer optimum relief from pain.

### *Heat Treatments*
- Take a lengthy, warm shower first thing in the morning after waking up to reduce morning stiffness
- Try utilizing a warm paraffin wax treatment system, which is available at a number of drug stores
- Soak yourself in a whirlpool or warm bath
- You can make a moist heat pad at home or get one from a drug store. If making one at home, place a wet wash cloth inside a freezer bag and heat it for one minute in a microwave. Wrap this hot pack inside a towel and position it over the area for relieving pain. Try this for 15 minutes.
- To soothe your painful and stiff joints, apply coconut oil and place that area under warm running water for a few minutes.
- You can even warm your clothes in a dryer before wearing them, or use an electric blanket when getting out of bed on cold days

### *Cold treatments*
- Wrap a bag of ice inside a towel and place it on the affected joints for a minimum of 10 minutes.
- Similarly, you can use a bag of frozen veggies and wrap a towel around it. This time of 'cold-pack' tends to conform around your joints.

## Enjoy the Benefits of Massage
A soothing massage is an excellent way of dealing with pain caused by arthritis. Massaging techniques can be used to soothe

sore muscles, particularly those that have been compromised as a result of flare-ups. Massage, regardless of whether it is conducted in a day spa or whether in a treatment room at your local physical therapy clinic, is definitely something that many people turn to in order to soothe sore muscles and joints, to reduce anxiety and to get them to sleep better.

The National Institute of Health's National Centre for Complementary and Alternative Medicine (NCCAM) states that massage is undoubtedly a popular and effective type of therapy used, with estimates showing that around 9 per cent of all Americans use it. However, until recently, not much was known as to why massages worked surprisingly well in reducing blood pressure, heart rate, anxiety and other health related issues.

However, the question is, is massaging safe for people with arthritis-like conditions such as pseudogout?

## Arthritis & Massage

Massaging, or getting someone to massage your muscles and joints has been linked to a significant reduction in pain associated with pseudogout. Regular massage can lead to improvements in your overall condition, including reduced pain and stiffness, increased range of motion, enhanced handgrip strength as well as an overall improvement in the performance of joints.

While the majority of research carried out on massage and its effects focuses on the general population, there has been an increase in the research aiming at people with arthritic conditions. For instance, a study carried out in 2006 study at the University of Medicine and Dentistry in New Jersey observed 68 adults who were suffering from knee osteoarthritis. Some of these participants received two Swedish massages every week for a period of eight weeks, compared to some who received none at all. The set of people who received the massage twice a week reported major improvements in stiffness, knee pain, function, walking and range of motion, according to the researchers.

Another research was carried out in the same year in Miami in which 22 adults with wrist arthritis were offered 4 weekly massages by a professional therapist while being taught how to massage their joints by themselves at home. A moderate-pressure massage was performed for 15 minutes in a day; however, this resulted in significantly reduced anxiety, pain, and an improvement in the strength of their grip as revealed by the pre and post therapy results.

Most individuals who wish to try out complementary therapies, such as massage, do in order to address neck and back pain, according to a report by NCCAM in 2007. Numerous studies confirm the fact that the massage for neck and back is really effective, including a study that was published back in 2011 in a journal called the Annals of Internal Medicine; this study observed the effectiveness of therapy (massage) on 401 people who had chronic back pain. According to the researchers, massage did indeed reduce the pain experienced by the participants, and the overall benefits lasted for around 6 months. It was also concluded that there was no difference in the type of massage performed as all worked fine.

Instead of the type of massage, what matters the most is the amount of pressure that is exerted during the massage therapy. According to therapists, light to moderate pressure is best for people with arthritis. A study was published in the International Journal of Neuroscience in 2010 that showed that by stimulating pressure receptors or the nerves beneath the skin, the pain reducing signals can be conveyed to the brain.

Laura McLaughlin, PhD, has been a part of this study and she explains:

*"The critical thing is using moderate pressure. Light pressure, just touching the surface of the skin or brushing it superficially, is not getting at those pressure receptors. Light pressure can be stimulating, not relaxing."*

## How Does Massage Work?

Even though a number of studies have shown that massage definitely reduces anxiety and pain in people with pseudogout, the question that remains is how does massage actually accomplish this?

According to research, massage tends to reduce the body's natural production of cortisol – a stress hormone – while enhancing the production of another hormone called serotonin. Serotonin has been found to enhance one's mood. To add to that, massage also lowers the production of substance P, a neurotransmitter, which is often linked to joint pain; this improves sleep and overall comfort level.

Researchers from Cedars-Sinai Medical Centre and the University of California's School of Medicine studied a group of 53 adults who received a single Swedish massage session, in which they found that the individuals' hormone levels as well as the white blood cells were affected, positively. For instance, a hormone called arginine-vasopressin, which can reduce blood pressure, was reduced, along with some inflammatory cytokines such as the IL-4 and the IL-10. The levels of Cortisol were also brought down as a result of the massage – however slightly. Christopher Moyer, a psychologist at the University of Wisconsin, says:

*"We know that massage reduces anxiety quite well and can reduce certain painful conditions rather well. But we don't know how those things are happening."*

In a study he published back in 2010, Moyer along with his colleagues figured out that massage therapy can reduce cortisol levels slightly. Nevertheless, this reduction is so slight that they concluded that the effects on levels of cortisol were not the main reason behind massage's ability to reduce stress and anxiety.

He added, *"Cortisol is a key stress hormone, but it doesn't mean that if we know a person's cortisol level, we know how much stress this person is having. Massage must be working in some other way."*

# Chapter 3: Eating Well

Due to the fact that pseudogout causes inflammation in joints, healthcare professionals recommend a few changes in the diet of the affected person to remove those foods that contribute to inflammation and add those foods that have anti-inflammatory properties.

This is precisely why great emphasis should be given to the foods you eat, particularly when you are trying to manage your pseudogout symptoms.

Fortunately, there are many kinds of foods that are extremely useful and effective in reducing inflammation and pain associated with pseudogout. A diet that is low in saturated fats and processed foods, along with being rich in vegetables, fruits, nuts, beans and fish can have surprising results on your overall heath, with noticeable effects on your medical condition.

In this chapter, you will find valuable guidelines that will help you choose the foods that are right for you.

## The Ultimate Diet

The following key foods should be made a regular part of your day-to-day diet. Science has proven the effectiveness of the following foods in lowering blood pressure, reducing the inflammation and pain of pseudogout flare-ups, while diminishing the chances of suffering from a stroke or heart attack.

### *Fish*

The Academy of Nutrition and Dietetics as well as the American Heart Association recommend at least 3-4 ounces of fish two times a week. Experts recommend more for people with arthritis, including pseudogout.

Some species of fish are extremely good sources of omega-3 fatty acids, which are known for their powerful inflammation-fighting abilities.

A study was carried out that identified, out of 727 women (post-menopausal), those that had the highest levels of omega 3. It was found that those women who consumed the greatest amount of omega 3 had low levels of inflammatory proteins called interleukin-6 and C-reactive protein (CRP).

Moreover, more recent studies have been carried out where researchers have focused on the use of fish oil supplements to see how effective they are in lessening inflammation, morning stiffness, as well as disease activity. Some of the patients who regularly use fish oil supplements have even been found to discontinue use of non-steroidal anti-inflammatory drugs (NSAIDs) without experiencing any flare-up pseudogout whatsoever.

**Best Sources:**

- Anchovies
- Herring
- Salmon
- Sardines
- Scallops
- Tuna

For those who do not want to eat fish, it is highly recommended that they at least take a fish oil supplement. It has been scientifically proven that taking between 600 and 1000 mg of fish oil eases tenderness, stiffness, swelling, and pain.

### *Nuts and Seeds*

Around a handful of seeds and nuts must be consumed on a daily basis. This adds up to around 1.5 ounces.

Nuts and seeds have a vital role to play in an inflammation-reducing diet. A study – conducted over a period of 15 years –was published in the American Journal of Clinical Nutrition and it found that people who ate the most amounts of nuts had an astounding 51 per cent lesser risk of dying from severe arthritis (or inflammatory disease, in general). While it is true that pseudogout is not a life-threatening condition, it does induce severe pain and may even immobilize an individual. Yet another study revealed that people with low Vitamin B6 levels (which are found in the majority of nuts) are more susceptible to oxidative damage and high CRP levels.

In addition, nuts contain anti-inflammatory monounsaturated fats that will reduce inflammation significantly.

Nuts are also rich in fibre and protein. Meanwhile, it is true that nuts are high in calories and fat, but it has been found that nuts actually promote weight loss due to the fact that their fats, protein, and fibre are satiating.

Nevertheless, unlike in the case of fish, more is not always the better when it comes to consuming nuts.

**Best Sources:**

- Almonds
- Pine nuts
- Pistachios
- Walnuts

Nuts can be mixed into all kinds of dishes and desserts.

### *Fruits and Vegetables*
It is recommended that people with pseudogout consume at least 9 or more servings of fruits and vegetables.

Fruits and vegetables are extremely rich in antioxidants, which are chemicals that help the body to defend itself from free radicals that are known to damage cells.

Our bodies produce around ten to fifteen oxidants each day. The process of oxidation can result in inflammation, thereby worsening various health conditions, such as causing pseudogout flare-ups.

The antioxidants found in fruits and vegetables effectively defuse these oxidants, thereby successfully protecting the body from the adverse effects of oxidants.

If you have pseudogout, you may want to consume more vegetables of the allium family that includes <u>garlic,</u> leeks, <u>onions,</u> and shallots. This is because these vegetables contain a compound called *diallyl disulphide* that effectively fights against corrupting protein enzymes found in individuals with arthritis.

**Best Sources:**

- Blackberries
- Blueberries
- Strawberries ←
- Kale
- Eggplant
- Bell Peppers ←
- Spinach ←
- Broccoli

## *Olive Oil*

Olive oil contains monounsaturated fat that is extremely heart-healthy and possesses anti-inflammatory properties. According to experts, as many as half the benefits of consuming olive oil actually come from olives, and not the oil itself. Olive oil is considered to be a delivery system for anti-oxidant compounds called polyphenols. The next time you dip your bread in olive oil and eat it, notice the slight scratching sensation at the back of your throat. This is a result of the phenolic compound – oleocanthal – that is a strong anti-inflammatory compound found in olive oil.

The compound has been found to inhibit activity of COX enzymes, thereby acting similarly to the action of ibuprofen. With that said, these enzymes help to dampen our body's inflammatory process as well as lowering the pain sensitivity.

**Best Sources:**

- Extra Virgin Olive Oil – this oil goes through considerably less processing and refining, therefore contains a greater number of nutrients than other, more refined versions.

## *Beans*

Beans contain a lot of fibre, which helps to bring down CRP, which is an indicator of the amount of inflammation found in the blood of a person. When found in high levels, CRP may indicate a mere infection or an RA.

Fibre is not the only thing in beans that helps them to combat inflammation. According to a recently published report in the Journal of Food Composition and Analysis, scientists studied the nutritional content found in ten most common varieties of beans. They identified a number of anti-inflammatory and anti-oxidant compounds, including genistein, quercetin, oleanolic acid, and soysapogenin.

Another reason that makes beans extremely beneficial, especially for people with pseudogout, is that they are a rich, cheap source of protein; they contain around 15 grams of protein per cup.

Protein plays a very important role in preventing the shrinkage of muscles as a result of inactivity and due to aging. The stronger muscles will help to keep your joints moving. Physical activity is crucial in pseudogout as well as other types of arthritis as you will see in the upcoming chapters.

Beans digest slowly due to their high fibre content, and thereby prevent your blood sugar levels from spiking up. Choose bean varieties that contain folic acid to gain an added advantage of a healthier heart. Some other immunity-boosting minerals found in beans include: iron, magnesium, potassium, iron, and zinc.

**Best Sources:**

- Small red kidney beans
- Red beans
- Garbanzo beans
- Black-eyed peas
- Pinto beans
- Black beans

## Nightshades: Should They Be Avoided?

Nightshade vegetables include tomatoes, eggplant, potatoes, and red bell peppers. Each of these vegetables is extremely capable of fighting diseases and provides a maximum amount of nutrition for the minimum amount of calories. However, they contain a chemical called *solanine.* This chemical is believed to be a culprit in making arthritis pain worse.

The Medical Director of the Centre for Integrative Medicine and Wellness Institute at the Cleveland Clinic says, concerning the effects of nightshades on arthritis, that there is no solid scientific evidence that links the possibility of the nightshade vegetables causing or increasing pain in arthritic patients. On the contrary, some experts state that this group of vegetables actually contains a powerful blend of nutrients that inhibits pain.

Eggplant, for instance, contains anti-inflammatory anthocyanins along with a decent quantity of fibre. All of this comes at a cost of only 35 calories for each cup.

Tomatoes contain an anti-oxidant called lycopene, which has been found to neutralize free radicals.

Red peppers, on the other hand, come loaded with vitamin C – a vitamin that boosts the human immune system. Potatoes are rich in potassium, which has a crucial role in controlling blood pressure, along with offering numerous other health benefits.

Not many people report any significant improvements in their symptoms when they avoid nightshade vegetables in their diets.

You should make them a part of your diet, and if you feel a flare up has resulted due to them, that is when you should eliminate them from your daily diet for a few days.

Only if you feel any improvement as a result of boycotting these vegetables should you avoid eating these vegetables as you are among those few who have an adverse effect from nightshade vegetables.

## The Link between Gluten-Free Diets and Joint Pain

There is a lot of talk these days concerning the benefits of gluten-free diets, with a great number of people claiming to benefit from such diets in terms of a reduction of digestive problems as well as in joint pain. While it is true that removing gluten from the diet can benefit those with celiac disease, it may not bring around the same benefits for those who do not suffer from this disease.

For those people who suffer from celiac disease, ingesting gluten tends to set off an inflammatory reaction in their small intestines. This damages the intestines' ability to effectively absorb nutrients from the food. With time, the poor absorption of minerals and vitamins leads to skin rashes, fatigue, or even osteoporosis (due to shortage of calcium).

Alessio Faranso, the director of the mucosal biology research centre at the University Of Maryland School Of Medicine in Baltimore, says:

*"The most accredited theory is that gut inflammation triggered by gluten causes the activation of T lymphocytes that can eventually migrate to joints, causing local inflammation and, therefore, joint pain. This theory is in line with the fact that celiac disease is now defined as a systemic disease that can affect any organ or tissue, including joints."*

The mechanisms involved in gluten sensitivity are currently under scrutiny. There are, however, certain reactions to ingestion of gluten that include bloating, diarrhoea, and in certain cases, joint pain that are almost the same as in celiac disease.

According to a dietician and a gluten-free diet expert at Celiac Disease Foundation and Gluten Intolerance Group, joint pain can surface in both the cases of gluten sensitivity and celiac disease.

If you think gluten is contributing to your joint pain, then you should consult a doctor and have a blood test to detect the presence of the disease. The results will reveal whether you need to follow a gluten-free diet or not.

## Omega-3 Fatty Acids: The Benefits

In order to understand why you should consume foodstuff containing omega-3 fatty acids, it is imperative to understand the benefits associated with them. Until recently, not many people were truly clear about the benefits of consuming omega-3 fatty acids. A study was carried out at Brigham and Women's Hospital in Boston, which revealed that these fatty acids actually convert into a type of compound that is almost ten-thousand times more potent than the original omega-3 fatty acids themselves.

These compounds consist of resolvins – which have a positive impact in lowering the inflammatory response in our bodies.

The normal inflammatory process in a healthy immune system repairs any damage while protecting the body from infections. However, in inflammatory conditions such as pseudogout, arthritis and others, the over-active immune response causes the degradation of tissues. Omega-3's conversion into highly effective compounds tends to halt this process, thereby switching off the factors that lead to inflammation.

It is not yet known how much omega-3 is required to fully optimize the body's omega-3 conversion process. The American Dietetic Association (ADA) recommends eating food instead of taking supplements to get the required omega-3. The best source of omega-3 is fish. Consume at least two servings of fish every week.

## Pseudogout Food Myths

There are many claims about certain foods that have the power to suppress or to deteriorate pain associated with pseudogout. There have been instances where individuals have claimed that certain foods aggravated their pain, such as after eating sugar, or that a patient has experienced lesser pain as a result of taking a few teaspoons of cider vinegar.

The question is: what is the truth behind such claims and how can you differentiate between science and myth?

It is important to understand and differentiate between what is true and what is not. This section will reveal some of the most common pseudogout-food and diet related myths.

### *Myth: A handful of raisins soaked in gin can provide pain relief*

When being processed, raisins are treated with sulfur dioxide gas in order to ensure that their color is preserved. Sulfur has been found to have a role to play in the health of joints. Around 25 years ago, a group of Russian researchers learnt that dimethyl sulfoxide had a positive effect in reducing destructive joint changes in rats.

One other research revealed whether or not the sulfur compound called methylsulfonylmethane has an effect on pain associated with osteoarthritis (OA).

At best, the results can be deemed inconclusive; however, such studies tend to feed the widespread belief that sulfur found in raisins actually has anti-inflammatory effects on these diseases.

As for the gin, juniper berries are the source used to make gin. These were indeed prescribed in the Middle Ages for their own self-supposed benefits – nothing has been proven about their anti-inflammatory properties.

**Bottom Line: Science has not yet provided any evidence that gin-soaked raisins actually reduce the pain or inflammation caused by pseudogout.**

### Myth: Consumption of cider vinegar alleviates pain

Some people claim that beta-carotene found in apple cider vinegar eliminates free radicals in our bodies. Free radicals are involved in damaging the human immune system. Nevertheless, the amount of beta-carotene found in cider vinegar is minute. If this approach really worked, anyone who ate carrots regularly would be completely free of pain associated with arthritis-type conditions.

Alternatively, there is a belief that joints tend to become stiff when acid crystals inside them harden. According to many, the vinegar is capable of dissolving these crystals and flushing them out of the body.

As a matter of fact, gout and pseudogout are the only types of arthritis that involve the buildup of crystals; and there is no scientific proof that cider vinegar can flush these out or reduce the pain linked with the condition. Supposing that the acid could break down the crystals, Irwin Rosenberg, a gastroenterologist explains:

*"You can't direct acid from your mouth to whatever part of the body you want."*

**Bottom Line: Apple cider vinegar should not be used as a medicine for treating or managing pseudogout.**

### Myth: Dairy products worsen pseudogout

A couple of years back, Dr Panush conducted a research where he put subjects with arthritis on dairy-free diets or on a placebo diet. The majority of those people who were put on a dairy-free diet fared no better than the people who were placed on placebo diets. The findings were published in Arthritis & Rheumatism in the year 1983.

As a matter of fact, researchers working at the University of Auckland in New Zealand found that dairy products protected against pseudogout. They revealed that the consumption of milk brings down the serum urate concentrations by almost ten percent, thereby reducing the chances of pseudogout development. This was published in the Annals of Rheumatic Diseases.

**Bottom Line: Dairy products might not be suitable for those who have some degree of intolerance to lactose. Apart from this, dairy products are in fact beneficial for people with pseudogout and other types of arthritis.**

*Myth: Nightshade vegetables worsen arthritis-type conditions*
Even though this has been discussed previously in this book, it is worth recalling due to the fact that this is among one of the most common myths circulating around the globe.

Vegetables such as eggplants, tomatoes, potatoes, and peppers fall under the banner of nightshade vegetables. All of these vegetables contain solanine – a chemical that has been considered to be a culprit in pain associated with arthritis. Nevertheless, no research has confirmed this claim at all.

On the contrary, the latest research actually suggests that these vegetables may actually help to diminish symptoms linked to numerous types of arthritis, including pseudogout and gout. The Journal of Nutrition revealed, early this year, that purple and yellow potatoes reduced the blood markers for inflammation in men.

Another research by Johnston County Osteoarthritis Project in NC, United States, revealed that individuals with high serum levels of a certain anti-oxidant (lutein) found in tomatoes were seventy-percent less likely to suffer from osteoarthritis.

**Bottom Line: Individuals with arthritis (including pseudogout) may benefit from consuming nightshades.**

*Myth: A raw food diet eases symptoms*
Finnish scientists reported in the British Journal of Rheumatology that a group of arthritic patients were put on a normal diet and one group was put on a raw vegan diet, which was complemented

with drinks rich in *lactobacilli* (bacteria that is supposedly good for the immune system and the gut).

Those who were placed on a raw diet reported to experience a greater reduction in their symptoms. Moreover, when they returned to their normal diets, which involved meat and cooked foods, their symptoms returned.

The positive effects of the raw foods were actually not apparent in something that the researchers termed 'objective measures of disease activity', which included pain at rest, morning stiffness, and pain during movement. Not only that, but half of those people who were on a raw diet began experiencing 'side-effects' of the diet, which included diarrhea and nausea, leading to them abandoning the experiment in advance.

**Bottom Line: It is a good idea to eat lots of uncooked vegetables and fruits as long as you consume them with just the right frequency so that the additional fiber does not lead to discomfort in your stomach. However, it is not clear as of yet that a major dietary change leading to a completely raw-diet is beneficial in managing pseudogout.**

*Myth: The more of red wine you drink, the better*
*"There are really interesting data on a compound in red wine resveratrol that show anti-inflammatory effects."* states Sharon Kolaninski, the director of the rheumatology fellowship program at the University of Pennsylvania School of Medicine in Philadelphia.

A study that was published in the Journal of Clinical Endocrinology and Metabolism constituted of only twenty individuals, supplements containing resveratrol, and no involvement of wine at all.

Even though it is clear that red wine, in small amounts, can actually bring about certain health benefits, such as protecting the heart and the body from food-related diseases, excessive

consumption can actually amplify the production of cytokines –
which contribute to inflammation.

**Bottom Line: It is crucial to consume red wine in moderation.
Women should drink no more than two glasses each day, and
men no more than three. Dr Kolasinki says:**

*"It would be taking it a little far to recommend more and more
red wine on the basis of that preliminary research."*

# Chapter 4: Losing Weight

Even though the majority of people understand the importance of maintaining a healthy weight for their well being, it can be quite a challenge for them to actually achieve their target weight due to a number of reasons. This has been proven by a study conducted out by the American Psychological Association (APA), which noticed that excess weight (being overweight or obese) is the number one health issue facing the US.

In spite of the fact that over 68 percent of all Americans fall in the category of being overweight or obese, the health problem can be solved. Losing as little as 5 or 10 pounds can bring about long-term health benefits.

It is crucial that you understand that losing weight is not a marathon regardless of whether you need to lose 10, 50, or even 100 pounds. It is also imperative to know that the benefits of shedding weight go beyond the physical appearance. It is considered to be a life-long process that you must continue in order to become healthier not only for yourself, but also for your family.

Losing weight is even more important for those who suffer from pseudogout and other forms of arthritis. This is because the weakening joints lose their capability to support excess weight, and a condition such as pseudogout can actually be more painful for overweight or obese people. With that said, let us start this chapter by talking about the benefits that can be gained by losing weight.

## Benefits of Losing Weight

Some of the benefits of losing weight are as follows:

### Reduced Pressure on Joints

A study published in Arthritis & Rheumatism in 2005 focused on overweight and obese individuals who had knee osteoarthritis and found that losing as little as a single pound of weight can remove approximately four pounds of pressure from their knees. Putting this in other words, by losing approximately 10 pounds of weight, you can take off 40 pounds of pressure off of the knees.

### Reduction in Pain and Inflammation

A 2010 study carried out by the University of Paris was published in the *Annals of Rheumatic Disease* and it revealed that weight loss can have significant effects in reducing pain, improving function and lowering inflammation levels within the body. The authors of a study called *Effects of Exercise and Physical Activity on Knee Osteoarthritis* also noted that physical activity, which helps in weight loss, can help by reducing pain as well as other symptoms of arthritis.

### Helps With Sleep Apnea

*"Weight losses of just 10 percent of a person's body weight (or about 20 pounds in those who weigh 200 pounds) have also been shown to have a long-term impact on sleep apnea ..."* says Rena Wing, a professor of psychiatry and human behavior at Brown University's Alpert Medical School. She is also the director of the Weight Control and Diabetes Research Center at The Miriam Hospital in Providence, Rhode Island.

The American Heart Association (AHA) reported that a reduction in obesity is the single, most effective factor that can protect a person from sleep apnea.

### Reduces the Risk of Developing Chronic Diseases

Data extracted from a study led by Centers for Disease Control and Prevention (CDC) showed that losing weight – even moderately – can reduce the risk of developing diabetes (type 2) by as much as 58-percent. It defined 'moderate weight loss' as shedding approximately 14 pounds.

Weight loss also brings down the risk of numerous diseases including cancer, while playing a crucial role in preventing and treating arthritis-related conditions.

### *Reduces the Risk of Cardiovascular Diseases*
Studies indicate that losing weight can quite effectively lower blood pressure, bringing it down into a healthy range. Additionally, eating healthily and carrying out regular exercise also lead to weight loss, and play a role in lowering cholesterol. Weight loss of as little as five to ten pounds can decrease blood pressure as well as the risk of suffering from cardiovascular diseases.

It is clear from the above benefits that losing weight plays a crucial role in the overall health of an individual. It is not only important to prevent dangerous diseases, but also helps arthritis (including pseudogout) patients better manage their condition.

## The Challenges of Weight-Loss Candidates
There are many challenges that individuals who are trying to lose weight have to face. It is important to fully understand these challenges in order to overcome them successfully.

## The Diet Killers
If your scale is stuck and refuses to budge towards the lower side, it is important to identify the underlying cause without blaming your willpower, or rather the lack of it. There can be a surprising number of things that can prevent you from losing weight, some of them we will cover in this section.

### *Snack Packs*
These 100-calorie snack packs found at grocery stores have a complicated psychology to them. They are based on the concept of 'unit bias', a term given to them by consumer scientists. This concept simply means that the bigger the size of a serving of any particular type of food, the more likely a person is to eat more of it. If the size of the *packaging* is reduced, people seem to think

that they would eat less; however, this does not stand true in the case of dieters.

According to a study by Arizona State University, non-dieters consumed lesser calories of M&Ms from a mini pack; however, dieters consumed about double the amount of calories when they ate out of snack packs instead of traditional packaging. The authors of this study wrote:

*"Consumers perceive the mini-packs to be diet food. For chronic dieters, this perceptual dilemma causes a tendency to overeat, due to their emotion-laden relationship with food."*

Putting this in simpler words, snack packs seem to give off an impression of being 'safer'; this is why dieters felt free consuming more M&Ms out of them.

### *Diet Soda*
Soft drinks are among some of the largest sources of calories in a typical American diet, and a number of studies that have been carried out on soda have linked them to weight gain. It has been found that even the calorie-free varieties are a culprit and cause weight gain. According to researchers, a single can of diet soda consumed each day can increase an individual's risk of getting obese by almost 41 percent. This was published in a journal called *Obesity.*

Sharon Fowler, a faculty associate in clinical epidemiology at the University of Texas Health Sciences Center, says:

*"We didn't prove that it causes weight gain, just that it's connected to it. One possibility, which we haven't studied yet, is that there's a chemical in diet soda that increases appetite."*

A number of dieticians point to yet another reason that causes diet soda drinkers to put on more weight: They consume soda in order to justify their poor food choices. As Tanya Zuckerbrot – a dietician based in New York – explains:

*"I've had clients tell me that they figured it was OK to have a cheeseburger and fries because their soft drink didn't contain calories."*

As far as soda is concerned, it is best that you swap it for water, seltzer or unsweetened iced tea. If you really cannot do without soda, only drink one can every other day.

### Having Too Many Choices

You may believe that having numerous types of food options would make you more satisfied; however, it is the opposite that is true. A study was carried out at the University of Pennsylvania where it was found that those people who were given a bowl containing 300 M&Ms with around 10 different colors consumed 43 percent more M&Ms as compared to the people who were given the same quantity of M&Ms but with only seven varieties of colors.

*"When you have fewer items, it's easier to grasp how much you're consuming,"* explains a clinical professor of Psychology at the same University, who is also an author of the famous *Complete BeckDiet for Life.*

Whenever possible, limit yourself to no more than 2 or 3 choices whenever you are eating at a buffet or a salad bar instead of tasting every single thing that is present. This way, you will also have a semblance of control over what you put on your plate – always opt for greener options, leaner protein and whole grains.

### Getting Tempted By Names

There's a reason why restaurants and food chains tend to give exotic names to their desserts, such as Chocolate Molten Lava Cake. These scrumptious sounding names really work – in their favor!

A study was conducted at the University of Illinois that found that when a simple piece of plain cake was named Black Forest Double Chocolate Cake, people found it to be more delicious and there was a greater chance that people would purchase it and eat it compared to when it was just called Chocolate Cake. On the other hand, researchers also found that when certain foods were termed 'healthy', people were less likely to buy it and believed that it did not taste good.

With that said, it is important that you keep an eye out for this phenomenon so that you can protect yourself from this trap. Just like you cannot judge a book by its cover, you cannot judge the taste of a particular food by its name.

### Eating at 'Healthy' Restaurants

There are numerous restaurants out there that claim to be a 'healthier' option; as a matter of fact, such restaurants can backfire particularly if you are not careful about what you eat there. People who eat at 'healthier' fast food chains, such as Subway, tend to eat more than people who go to 'normal' food chains such as McDonalds. This was proven by a study conducted at Cornell University.

*"When people think a type of food is good for them, they think that it can do no wrong, so they don't pay attention to their portion sizes and don't check to see how many calories they're consuming,"* says Blatner, who is the author of a famous best seller *The Flexitarian Diet.*

The best approach you can adopt is to do a little research before you head out to eat. Visit the website of the restaurant and dig for some nutritional information so you are well aware in advance what you are eating. This will help you make an informed decision when actually at the restaurant. When aiming for healthy food choices, you should aim for no more than 500 calories and saturated fat less than 6 grams.

### Enjoying a Free Day

One of the most destructive things you can do that will disrupt your diet is to treat yourself with an 'off' day – a day where you eat whatever you feel like irrespective of your healthy diet.

If you had succeeded in losing some weight, eating like this on weekends or 'off' days will actually promote weight gain and you may end up right where you started.

Due to the fact that it is important to give yourself a certain amount of leeway, give yourself bonus 150 calories each day so that you do not feel suffocated by your diet. These calories are enough to satisfy your cravings every now and then; however, they are not as many as to affect your health in a negative manner.

## Dangers of Yo-Yo Dieting

Once you have shed the excess weight, it can be difficult to keep it from coming back. However, according to the latest research, it has been found that it is even more challenging for middle-aged women to prevent re-gaining of weight. They have to be extra cautious; otherwise they may experience what is called yo-yo dieting.

A study was carried out by researchers at the Wake Forest University School of Medicine in which they evaluated 78 individuals considered to be abdominally obese. These individuals were menopausal women who had shed around 12 percent of their overall body weight as a result of adhering to a low calorie diet.

One year after they had ended the low calorie diet, as many as 76 percent of women regained some of the weight they had shed. In general, the women on diets had lost twice the amount of fat as compared to muscle. Nonetheless, they still regained the weight after a period of one year, and that too almost four times the amount of fat.

The researchers did not focus on how the weight gain affected their health; or the number of times the individuals had lost or gained weight. What they did realize is that losing muscle mass can be especially problematic for adults because this is precisely what can reduce their physical mobility. This can cause problems in day-to-day activities such as climbing the stairs, particularly for middle-aged women.

Thus, the outcome of the research was that middle-aged women –
particularly those that have arthritis – need to be more cautious
and ensure that they maintain their muscle mass when they are
regaining weight or dieting. Jon Giles, assistant professor of
medicine at Columbia University's College of Physicians &
Surgeons, states:

*"Chronic inflammation causes muscle loss in those patients and
since they're already starting out with low muscle mass, they
should emphasize maintaining that muscle during weight loss
even more."*

Loss of muscle can further deteriorate arthritis and associated
conditions such as pseudogout. This is because muscle is needed
to support the damaged joints.

In order to minimize muscle loss when following a diet, or if you
feel as if you are regaining weight after ending a diet, it would be
a wise idea to consume foods that are rich in protein. Exercise
will also help immensely alongside eating high-protein foods.

## Identifying and Managing Eating Triggers
You may be at the annual family reunion and trying so hard to
stay away from all the delicious food spread out on the table, but
then you spot the apple pie and just cannot stop thereafter. There
are certain triggers that can make us overeat or eat foods that are
unhealthy for us.

It is crucial for people with pseudogout and other forms of
arthritis to ensure that they keep their weight within the healthy
range. A well-managed weight not only helps to keep
inflammation at its lowest, but also makes exercising easier while
reducing the pressure exerted on joints. It also reduces the risk of
developing a cardiovascular disease.

This is precisely why it's important for you to identify and learn
to manage the triggers that can lead you to overeat. Some of the
most common pitfalls are as follows, along with the advice on
how you can overcome each of them.

### Family Pressure

Family pressure can be intense when it comes to food. Your grandmother may force you to eat your favorite apple pie that she baked especially for you.

The solution to eliminate this trigger is to initiate a direct conversation whenever possible. There is no better way to convey your message than clearly defining your calorie goals.

### Social Snacking

You may be at a party where you are making multiple trips to the snack table like everyone else there is doing.

This is a mirroring effect that is common at parties. When you see other people eating and having a great time, you are encouraged to do the same.

The solution to this is to sit down. When you tend to move about more at parties and gatherings, you can easily lose track of what you are eating. Another way to counter this is by eating a healthy, wholesome meal before you go to the party. This will make you less inclined to indulge in whatever is available. It may also effectively keep you from consuming too many alcoholic drinks.

### Great Deals

You may be tempted to select a deal that includes an appetizer, entrée, and a dessert at a fixed price that is much lower than what it would cost you if you were to order each item separately.

People want something that gives them the most out of their money; and marketers utilize this technique to distort our understanding of what is healthy for us.

This is a trigger that makes it necessary for us to slightly modify our mindset. Learn to appreciate the fact that budget-friendly foods generally lead to poor health and a gain in weight in the long run. Whenever you feel tempted to select such a deal, ask yourself whether you really need it – do not forget to consider the combined nutritional values of the deal.

### Emotional Eating

Some people tend to eat a lot when they are feeling sad. This means that they may eat a whole bag of chips or other unhealthy snack and they may not realize how harmful this can be for their health.

As humans, we tend to eat things based on our mood. Learn to understand what moods lead to unhealthy eating and try to come with alternatives that you can eat or drink when in that particular mood. For instance, the next time you're feeling a little blue, take a hot bath, sipping on a cup of warm tea instead of munching snacks.

### Cleaning Your Plate

Whenever you order something at a restaurant, the size of the serving seems to be 'fine'; after all, you chose something from the 'healthy menu'.

It is not easy to figure out the right size of a serving. According to a number of studies carried out on this, it has been found that we are generally poor guessers when it comes to determining the amount of fat, calories, sugar, or sodium in a meal. Do not forget the fact that a serving size and a portion size are two different things. The former refers to the recommended size of a food portion; the latter, on the other hand, is the actual amount of food you have opted to eat – it can be bigger or smaller than the recommended serving size.

The best way to overcome this habit is to educate yourself. There are many restaurants out there that provide nutritional information on their website. You can always refer to this information prior to heading out for your meal. You obviously do not have to waste good food, simply eat a portion that seems appropriate for you, and take the rest home in a take-home bag.

## 10 Easy Ways to Reduce Caloric Intake

Reducing the number of calories you take in does not necessarily mean that you are going on a particular diet. Even slight changes in your life can make a huge difference in reducing your calories.

For instance, controlling the size of your portions and reducing the time you spend watching TV can help you to lose weight quickly and effectively.

Here are 10 tips to help you bring down the number of calories you consume on a daily basis:

### *Cut down on sugar*
Use artificial sweetener instead of sugar in your tea or coffee. You won't notice the difference in terms of taste, but you will definitely save yourself from gaining a few pounds.

For each cup, you will save around 15 to 30 calories.

### *Choose light mayonnaise*
Light mayonnaise contains almost half of all the calories found in the 'real' mayo. Just like the artificial sweetener, you wouldn't notice any changes in terms of taste, but will be limiting yourself from gaining extra pounds.

You will cut your calories into half by switching from normal mayonnaise and to the lighter alternatives.

### *Select sugar-free cocoa*
The regular cocoa mixes contain around 120 calories. Sugar-free varieties, on the other hand, comprise of much lesser calories per serving – ranging from between 60 and 90.

### *Select light syrup*
Light syrup contains half the calories as compared to traditional syrup varieties. You will save around 50 calories per serving.

### *Opt for a frozen fudge pop*
As compared to milk chocolate's caloric amount, a no-sugar added frozen chocolate pop would have only 40 calories. If you want to treat your sweet tooth, why not choose this option?

After all, you will be saving around 110 calories!

### Reduce the size of your tortilla

Reduce the size of your flour tortilla from 10 inches down to 6 inches – and choose the corn version. A 10-inch flour tortilla typically contains 220 calories, whereas a 6-inch corn alternative would satisfy you in 90.

### Use soy crumbles instead of ground beef

Soy crumbles contain around 90 calories as compared to the 220 calories of ground beef for a 3-ounce serving.

This will save you 130 calories.

### Refine your drink

Instead of using tonic water or regular soda in your drinks (150 calories), use sparkling water or diet soda (0 calories).

You will cut down on 150 calories.

### Reduce your steak portions

Reduce the size of your steak from a 6-ounce serving (320 calories) to a 3-ounce serving. Add salad to make it an overall healthier meal.

You will save yourself from around 160 calories.

### Light cheese strings

If you cannot resist your temptation to eat cheese, select the light string variety, which will save you 30 calories.

# Chapter 5: Protecting Your Joints

Due to the nature of arthritis and arthritis-related medical conditions such as pseudogout, it is very important that you take measures to protect your joints from degradation and further damage.

This chapter will provide you with valuable guidelines and information on this matter.

## Top Ways To Protect Your Joints

*Avoid Neck Pain* – Attach document holders at an eye-level near your computer monitor and use hands-free telephone headsets to reduce the chances of straining your neck muscles.

*Compute Comfortably* – Make sure that your upper body section is at a distance of between 20 and 26 inches from the computer's monitor. The top of the monitor should be at a line even to the top of your head when it is in the neutral position. Make sure that your arms hang at ease on your sides; the elbows should be make right angles while your wrists should be relaxed when you are typing.

*Avoid Wearing High Heels* – Unless you have to wear high heels for a living, you can certainly live without them. According to experts, a mere three-inch heel imposes 7 times more stress than a 1-inch heel. Heels tend to put a lot of stress on your knees and will increase your risk of developing osteoporosis.

*Sit and Stand* - Sitting or standing continuously for prolonged periods of time is not good for your feet. Whenever possible, change your position from one to the other in order to prevent locking in one position.

*Allow Your Wrists to Rest* – Get yourself a wrist rest for use when operating a computer or make yourself one using two strips of bubble-wrap packing material and taping it together. Ensure that the bottom strip is wider than the one on the top; also, do not forget to tape the excess portion to your keyboard's bottom. This will ensure that your wrists extend outwards comfortably.

***Handle Heavy Loads Properly*** – To make the handling of heavy loads easier, utilize your strongest muscles and joints to reduce the stress on smaller joints and muscles. This can be accomplished by spreading the load over a larger area. Use both of your palms when lifting or carrying items instead of just using the hands.

Hold the items closer to your body as this would impose lesser stress on your joints. To ensure the safety of your joints, whenever possible, slide objects instead of lifting them.

***Make Efforts to Reduce Weight*** – We have already discussed the importance of losing weight for those people who suffer from pseudogout or other forms of arthritis. Not only will this make you look better, but you will also feel a lot better as well. Every pound you gain tends to put around 4 times more stress on your joints, particularly the knees.

Losing weight even to the slightest extent will take the load off your knees considerably. According to research, losing around 11 pounds can improve your joint's health as well as reduce the risk of developing osteoarthritis by as much as 50 percent.

 ***Visualize Your Portion Sizes*** – It is crucial that you eat the right sized portions in order to maintain a healthy weight, which would lessen the load exerted on your joints. Make visual comparisons when it comes to portion sizes. For example, a 3-ounce serving of meat should be around the size of your palm; a serving of dairy, let us assume - 2 oz. of cheese – would be like a pair of dominoes; on the other hand, a serving of vegetables amounting to one cup would be around your fists' size.

***Turn Off the Tele*** - Television has a really important role in keeping us sedentary. This tends to slow down our metabolism and also makes us eat more than we should be eating. Read a book or put on your sneakers and go out to jog!

***Build Strong Bones*** – Increase the amount of calcium you take in, because a calcium-rich diet will keep your bones strong and sturdy while significantly lowering your risk of developing osteoporosis. There are numerous sources of calcium besides milk, such as broccoli, yoghurt, figs, kale, salmon, as well as calcium supplements.

***Avoid the Drive Thru*** – You must avoid eating food at fast food restaurants. However, if you really have to eat something there, try to choose something that is relatively healthier. For instance, go for grilled meat instead of fried meat. Add tomato and lettuce to your burger or sandwich. Stay away from mayonnaise. In the place of fries, get a salad. Water is the best option when it comes to beverage.

***Make Your Diet Colorful*** – Add various fruits and vegetables to ensure that you get a wide variety of nutrients, including fiber, antioxidants and a lot of phytochemicals.

***Linger At The Salad Bar*** - Eating vegetables that are normally found in a plain tossed salad in a salad bar, such as Bibb lettuces, romaine, spinach, broccoli, parsley and kale, can significantly reduce bone loss that occurs with age, according to research. This is because these vegetables are rich in calcium; however, do not spoil it all by topping them with dressings.

***Become Supplement Savvy*** – Glucosamine is a supplement that is made out of the shells of lobster, crab and shrimp. This supplement has been found to reduce joint pain and relieve stiffness, especially in people who are suffering from pseudogout our other forms of arthritis. Some studies even suggest that the supplement has the ability to repair the damaged cartilage.

***Eat Lots of Fish*** – Cold-water fish contain rich quantities of Omega-3 fatty acids. These can help to keep your bones and joints in optimal health. As a matter of fact, some studies have shown that Omega-3 fatty acids can actually lessen the pain and reduce inflammation in stiff joints in individuals with arthritis. While you may not have the time to grill fish each day, you may want to get fish oil capsules to supplement your diet.

***Munch on Healthy Food*** - Keep vegetables and fruits, such as carrot, broccoli florets, melon cubes, and pepper slices and melon cubes, in an easily-reachable position in your refrigerator so that you can reach out to them when you feel like snacking.

***Maintain A Food Journal*** – You can increase your chances of sticking to your plan of eating well and exercising well. Keep a record of what you do each day as it will motivate you to go on.

***Break Your Meals*** – Rather than eating 2 or 3 large meals every day, try to spread your food intake by eating smaller meals throughout each day. According to research, eating smaller meals throughout the day can increase the metabolism rate and help the body to function more efficiently.

***Cut Down on Caffeine*** – Even though caffeine does give you that much-needed boost in the morning, avoid going for second and third cups as excessive caffeine intake can weaken the bones.

***Take Vitamins Regularly*** – A multivitamin is a great way to supplement your diet in order to gain the necessary vitamins and minerals that you may be lacking. To make your body strong, make sure you are getting sufficient quantities of Calcium, Vitamin C, Vitamin E, Vitamin K, and folic acid.

***Head Out To The Great Outdoors*** – You will not only be able to relax by breathing fresh air, but you will also get the chance to observe nature. You will get a lot of opportunities to burn those extra calories while you have fun. Take gardening, for instance. Other types of yard work provide other ways to tone up your arms, legs, and other muscles throughout your body. Your joints will remain active, something that is necessary for their health.

*Plunge into the Water* - From jogging to strength training to aerobic classes, aquatic exercises enable a person to do all the exercises that you love to do; however, there is an added advantage. All these activities can be performed in the water with much lesser stress on the joints!

*Go Hiking* – Find the spots that you love and head out at least 3 times a week. Hiking is an excellent activity that burns calories, builds denser bones, and strengthens muscles while you enjoy appealing scenery and get immersed into nature.

*Warm Up* – Never hit the gym, the trails, or the pool without warming up first! Warming yourself up is just like warming up your car during the winter months. To ensure that you perform as smoothly as possible, and to make sure that your joints are ready to take on the stress imposed by these activities, you have to start slow and allow yourself at least 5 minutes of preparation time.

*Go Comfortable, Not Fashionable* - Shoes aren't only supposed to look good; they should be extremely comfortable. Look for shoes that are supportive, flexible, and rounded/squared at the toes so you can move them around. A shoe that has a rubber sole provides more cushioning. Make sure you select shoes that are bendable at your foot's ball of your foot.

*Monitor Your Health* – After you exercise, monitor your health, particularly how you feel. If your joints continue to ache for more than 2 hours after you finish exercising, then they are definitely trying to tell you that something is not right. You may want to make your exercise routine less intense.

*Stretch Yourself* – Stretching can do wonders for your whole body. Stretching is not just about warming up before workouts. Whatever you are doing throughout your day, take breaks in between and stretch yourself. This is particularly important if you have a desk job where you sit for several hours straight, possibly working on a computer.

***Visit a Yogi*** – Yoga has been the hottest trend for several thousand years (you read that right!). Yoga, along with numerous exercises such as Tai Chi or Pilates are famous for strengthening the mind and body connection; enabling a person to get in shape while also getting the mind to relax. These exercises can also make your joints and muscles stronger while reducing or even eliminating stress.

***Bulk Up*** - Strength training, undoubtedly, is an effective way to enhance your metabolism. According to research, it has also been found that lifting weights makes the bones denser and helps the muscles to get stronger, particularly those that protect joints and stabilize them.

***Build Abs of Steel*** - Strong abs play a crucial part in enhancing your overall core balance and strength. The latest studies have shown that the balance and strength of your core are important to prevent falls and to protect the joints from any kind of damage.

***Brace Yourself*** - Use wrist, elbow, and joint braces to prevent them from any injury. Not only this, but these 'guards' will also reduce the load imposed upon your joints. Ask your healthcare professional if these braces can ease off some of the stress from your joints, and perhaps make movement easier for you.

***Get a Trainer*** – Why not sign up for consultation with a professional trainer? A professional can guide you on what exercises are safe for you, and what activities you should be avoiding. If you exercise incorrectly, you can cause undue damage to your joints.

***Avoid Stomping Your Feet*** – According to research, exercises that involve pounding, such as step aerobics, kickboxing, and the like, can actually be more stressful for your joints. Instead of performing these, go for low-impact activities such as swimming and cycling. The latter exercises offer you the same kind of calorie burning benefits, minus the pain and stress.

*Up Your Range* – Range-of-motion exercises, such as stretching and any others that increase your range, are an excellent way to keep your ligaments and muscles strong and flexible. Add some weights and you will be able to tone up your muscles too!

*Soak Up* – Soothe your aching joints and muscles by soaking in a warm bath right after you exercise. You have worked hard, go right ahead and treat yourself to a warm bath, without any guilt whatsoever.

*Write Your Way To Fitness* – Keep a journal in which you write about your feelings, deepest fears, and frustrations. This will bring everything into perspective. It will also enable you to look back and cherish your successes and victories. Some people have found that writing down their feelings can actually reduce pain to a certain extent.

*Enjoy a Massage* – A massage can be very effective in relieving muscle tension and can reduce fatigue significantly. Once in a while, get a massage from a professional or learn how to do it yourself. It is generally a good idea to get a massage after a stressful week at work. Some types of massage, such as the Swedish massage, give emphasis to improving the function of joints and muscles.

*Give Yourself Time Off* – Take time off from work and let yourself go on a vacation, preferably somewhere away from home and work. Don't get caught up in planning an expensive vacation to an island; just head out and break your routine. Stress and pain have a strong relation; don't let this relation thrive.

*Learn to Say No* – While this may be difficult at first, you will eventually begin to understand that it is for your own good. When you say no to others and to certain activities, you get additional time to yourself; time which you can use to relax and let your joints take a break. You can also exercise, meditate, and eat healthy in your free time!

*Soak Before You Sleep* – Taking a warm bath before you go to bed can alleviate muscle tension, reduce pain in the joints, and allow you to sleep well.

*Enjoy Heat Therapy* – Heat therapies provide an excellent way to ease pain and stiffness. Try warm showers, whirlpools, heated pools, microwaveable heat packs, and warm compresses.

*Utilize Cold Packs* – A cold pack can reduce pain, sore spots, and swelling. You can make a cold pack by wrapping up ice in a towel. You can even use a bag of frozen vegetables to quickly and easily reduce swelling. Try rubbing ice on your joint and see if it helps reduce pain in your particular case.

*Rub Analgesics* – Topical analgesics can help in cases of mild pain. Counter irritants, capsaicin, or salicylates can be really helpful in alleviating pain.

*Visit Your Doctor* - Visit your healthcare professional at least once a year for a routine check-up. Request a thorough examination of your joints and ask for advice on how you can reduce the daily wear and tear on them. It's always a good idea to learn self-management techniques when it comes to your joints, and of course, overall health.

*Reveal All Your Medications* - Make sure you tell your physician about all the medications that you may be taking, both over-the-counter and prescription. Tell him or her about any nutritional supplements that you may be taking. This is very important as certain medicines and supplements can have adverse effects with each other.

## Knee Support Braces

When Rex Benham, a famous US Racquetball player, was informed by his doctor that he required complete knee replacement surgery, he thought that his days as a racquetball player would come to an end. However, just five years later, Rex

Benham played in the National USA Racquetball Tournament without having any surgery whatsoever. He said:

*"I am almost always pain-free and walk and play without a limp."*

The credit for this goes to his quadriceps-strengthening routine, and to the knee brace that he used to relieve the pain associated with arthritis.

Some of the most well documented benefits of wearing knee braces for arthritis-like conditions, such as osteoarthritis and pseudogout are like the cases of Rex Benham; their cartilage damage had been confined to the inner compartment of their knee, according to Martin Leland, an orthopedic surgeon at the Department of Surgery at the University of Chicago.

*"The unloader brace pushes the knee back into its normal alignment and puts more of the force to the outside compartment and less on the damaged inside compartment so the knee feels better,"* says Leland.

There are three other ways in which a brace can help people who have arthritis in their knee:

### *Allows Ligaments to Heal*
When medial collateral ligament (MCL) injuries are concerned, a hinged knee brace can be prescribed by your healthcare provider. This brace will provide the essential support needed for the healing process. Anterior Collateral Ligament tears usually require surgery. In these cases, a drop lock hinged brace may be recommended by a physician, this locks the knee to make the knee immobile, or it may also be used to unlock the knee for recovery following a surgery.

### *Relieves Kneecap Pain*
When softness or weakness of cartilage below the kneecap induces pain, a Neoprene brace with a cutout for a kneecap may keep the bone in its correct place and alleviate pain. It should also allow you exercise comfortably in order to strengthen your

quadriceps. You can get these braces at sporting goods stores or pharmacies.

### *Boosts Confidence*

A lot of people have reported getting relief from pain when they used a neoprene sleeve-type brace. These braces can also be bought at sporting goods stores and pharmacies. According to experts, these help by providing compression and warmth; this, in turn, may reduce swelling. One of the main benefits, however, is psychological. Mat Holland, the manager of physical therapy at the Methodist Center for Sports Medicine in Houston, Texas, says:

*"It gives you a feeling of support and a reminder to be more careful of that knee when you're physically active."*

## A Few Steps to Prevent Falls

As you age, the consequences of a fall can be far more severe than before.

According to an estimate by the Centers for Disease Control and Prevention (CDC), around one-third of all people who are over the age of 65 fall; one out of ten of all people who fall require hospitalization.

Age is not the only factor; in fact, the scenario becomes worse when an individual has arthritis. Susan Avent, a nurse at the Duke University Hospital in NC, says:

*"Mobility in the patient with arthritis is often altered or limited, contributing to problems with balance. Patients with arthritis may suffer increased pain, often requiring the use of pain medications, which may further alter mobility."*

Slower reflexes, reduced strength, and reduced awareness of one's surroundings increase the problem.

However, even with all those factors, falls don't have to occur in your case. Here are some guidelines that will help to prevent falls and any fall-related injuries.

### *Avoid Multitasking when walking*

Multitasking while walking affects a person's ability to identify the situation where a fall becomes imminent. When you are walking, try to focus only on that so you have a better awareness of your surroundings and are placing your feet firmly and steadily as you take each step forward. This becomes more important when walking up or down the stairs.

### *Exercise*

Water workouts, Tai chi, and walking all increase your strength while enhancing your coordination, flexibility, and balance. The Arthritis Foundation in the US offers programs and activities to help you with the three qualities mentioned above.

### *Get Your Eyes Tested*

Identify and treat any vision problems before they get any worse. This will help you see better for longer!

### *Consider Your Medications*

There are some medicines that cause dizziness or drowsiness, and you should be extremely careful when moving about after consuming them. It is best that you take such medications right before you go to sleep, unless otherwise stated by the doctor. In the latter case, minimize your movement and find an activity that you can do while you remain seated.

### *Make Your Home Safe*

Clean up all the clutter on the floor and secure rugs and place mats (non-slip) in tubs and showers. Get the top edge of the steps painted to make them stand out.

### *Choose the Right Shoes*

High heels can almost always ruin your balance, particularly when you are suffering from arthritis/pseudogout. Floppy slippers can make you trip while brand-new shoes may feature slippery soles. Choose your shoes wisely! Preferably, you should wear shoes that grip the floor properly as this will reduce your chances of falling tremendously.

### Know Where Your Pets Are
Small dogs and cats can get underfoot very easily, while big dogs can knock you over. Researchers at the CDC have learned that pets are responsible for causing as many as 86,600 falls every year; people who are over the age of 75 are most likely to get injuries such as a broken bone.

### Reorganize
From clothing to pantry items to dishes, keep all those things that you need on a regular basis in a well-organized way. It would be best if you keep such things in a place where you do not have to climb up (such as in the case of cupboards). The more organized and easily accessible your things are, the less likely you are to face any problems in locating them.

## The Number 1 Cause of Falls: Poor Balance
A recent study has revealed that the most common reason behind falls in older people is poor balance (incorrect weight shifting), and not trips or slips. Falling down usually results in severe injury and often leads to hospitalization; it is also responsible for over 90 percent of all wrist and hip fractures in people over the age of 65.

Researchers, in an attempt to better understand the causes of falls, analyzed videos from numerous public areas, such as hallways, dining rooms, and lounges. They published their study in The Lancet this October. They learned that in as many as 41 percent of the cases, individuals were incapable of getting in a stable position when rising up from a seated position, or they could not stop their momentum (forward) after taking wrong step. They also found that the possibility of falling was almost as high when people lowered themselves into seats or when standing and being bumped by something or someone. This finding nullified the previous belief that people could only fall when they were walking.

The second most common reason behind a fall is tripping, and it remains to be a critical factor due to the fact that tripping causes around one-fourth of all falls. People often stumble and one of their feet collides with the other, thereby tripping them. This is more likely when they are turning. Other obstacles also cause them to trip, such as the leg of a table or a chair, or any items that may be littered on the floor.

*"There's an opportunity there for improved environmental design. One thought is to select furniture so there's a single central flaring support that provides for stability but removes the tripping hazard."* says Robinovitch.

Some of the falls were also a result of a person not wearing assistive devices when they were supposed to be wearing them. John FitzGerald, who is an associate clinical professor of medicine at the division of rheumatology at the University of California's David Geffen School of Medicine in Los Angeles, states that the findings can be really helpful for patients with arthritis-related conditions.

*"If [people] have arthritis of the lower extremities, they can have an abnormal gait that can throw them off balance and make them more susceptible to falls. And some arthritis medicines can further increase the risk of falls – specifically [opioid] pain relievers,"* he explains.

According to him, if a family member or yourself have fallen already or have come close to falling down for one reason or the other, they should consult a doctor to determine whether or not there is an underlying issue that may be causing you to lose balance or lack of coordination.

Using assistive devices, reviewing medication, and correcting any orthotics abnormalities can also bring down the risk level.

Additionally, it is crucial that you pay attention to the environmental hazards around you. For instance, ensure that you have sufficient lighting as well as handrails installed along the staircase. Meanwhile, it is imperative that you remove any hazards that may be lying on the floor. You may also want to enroll yourself for some resistance-training exercises to increase your balancing abilities, strength and flexibility; this is quite important particularly for upper arms as they can help you break a fall.

He explains, *"There are three essential abilities related to falls. One is the ability to safely move about without losing your balance. The others are the ability to recover balance by taking a step or grasping a nearby object, and then, if a fall does occur, the ability to protect yourself and land safely."*

There are numerous factors that are involved in the way massage may ease stiffness, pain, and anxiety. The exact mechanism that comes into action is still being investigated. For instance, a more relaxing sleep which results from massage therapy can help reduce arthritis-related pain.

## The Best Forms of Massage for Arthritis Conditions

If you are looking for the right type of massage to alleviate your arthritis pain, stiffness, and other symptoms, it is crucial that you contact your physician or a rheumatologist before you actually start your massage therapy.

There are techniques that involve the exertion of strong pressure to sensitive areas of joints and tissues. In addition, it can be difficult to move limbs into certain positions for someone who has damaged joints as a result of arthritis.

It is imperative that you exercise extreme caution when planning to try massage therapy in the following cases:

- Damaged / eroded joints due to arthritis
- Flare-ups of inflammation, skin rash or fever
- Severe osteoporosis

- High blood pressure
- Varicose veins

According to a physical therapist:

*"It's always a good idea to get the thumbs up or down from a doctor if you are having even the slightest worry about using massage for your condition. It's also very important to tell the therapist if you are experiencing pain or if you are uncomfortable with the work that he/she is doing. A good therapist will want feedback on what you are feeling during the session."*

Always make sure that you talk to your therapist well before the session is conducted to inform him or her of your arthritis. You should tell them which parts of your body have been affected.

In turn, therapists need to be careful and very cognizant as they have a long list of contraindications for massage in their minds.

The goals for massage will vary, depending on why you want to undergo massage therapy. You might be interested in the soothing effects of massage that reduce stress and anxiety as a result of arthritis; on the other hand, you may be looking to relieve your pain and stiffness on your joints. Talk freely with your therapist to let them know what you seek so that they can perform the ideal type of massage for your individual needs.

Most important of all, massage must make your pseudogout pain and the associated stiffness feel better and not worse. It is simple; if it hurts, don't do it.

Don't forget that massage is not medicine; it's a therapy to help you better manage your condition by reducing or eliminating pain, stiffness, and other symptoms associated with your medical condition. Thus, you should be enjoying the experience rather than despising it. Good communication with your health care provider and the physical therapist will guarantee optimum results.

## Acupuncture

Acupuncture has been around for 2000 years; however, it is only recently that it has become mainstream. According to research, acupuncture may have the potential to treat osteoarthritis, pseudogout, and rheumatoid arthritis.

The theory of acupuncture relates to an essential energy of life called qi (pronounced as chee). This energy is believed to flow through the body along twenty different, invisible channels called the meridians. Whenever the natural flow of this energy gets blocked or gets out of balance, pain or an illness occurs.

Acupuncturists, by stimulating these 'meridians', can correct the flow of the energy. Tim Rhudy, when talking to his patients, explained that the science of acupuncture can reduce pain by *"untying muscular straitjackets, releasing spasmed, tight, shortened muscles to their resting state."* Tim Rhudy is a licensed acupuncturist at Cleveland Clinic.

It is also believed to help regulate your body's nervous system. The nervous system plays a crucial role in stimulating the production and release of natural endorphins – chemicals that fight pain.

Acupuncture also helps the body by pinpointing where the health problems actually are. Whenever you get a cut on your hand, your body's natural response is to send help to the affected area. Similarly, as soon as a needle is entered in to the affected point, the body focuses on that area, thus boosting the healing factors in that region.

Acupuncture also tends to alter a person's perception of pain, as Rhudy says:

*"Brain magnetic resonance imaging shows that deep needling of acupuncture points deactivates the part of the brain that deals with our perception of pain."*

Here is some research regarding acupuncture:

- **Rheutamoid Arthritis (RA)** - A latest study from China reveals that traditional acupuncture & electroacupuncture can reduce tenderness significantly. This includes all of the 36 participants of the study who underwent the treatment, regardless of whether they had traditional acupuncture or the electroacupuncture. A total of 20 sessions over a 10 week period were conducted in which needles were inserted to a depth of between 10 and 20 mm; they were left their for 30 minutes.
- **Osteoarthritis (OA)** - A German study, comprising of 304,674 people with OA in their knee, received 15 acupuncture sessions along with their usual medical care. At the end of the study, it was found that they had reduced pain and stiffness. Their ability to function more effectively had increased, while the quality of life also went up. These improvements were evident immediately after the 3-month course of acupuncture was completed and the benefits lasted for a minimum of another three months. Thus, the outcome of this study was that acupuncture can improve OA.

## Getting Started with Meditation

Meditation comprises of numerous practices of relaxation and focused thinking. Regardless of what meditation technique you try out, the ultimate goal is to build coping strategies, boost your positive thinking, and eventually reduce anxiety and pain due to pseudogout.

It may be that you have tried it once, say a few sessions, but 2 minutes might have felt like 2 hours. In addition, after a 20-minute session, you might have felt the same: the same to-do list that just keeps piling up.

It is important to note that stress, anxiety, and depression have an impact on how you feel physically. These things reduce the body's ability to heal itself as it weakens the immune system.

This is the last thing that you would want particularly when you are trying to reverse the symptoms of pseudogout, and other arthritis conditions.

You are not alone when it comes to dealing with stress & anxiety. There are many people who are looking for ways to get rid of the excessive thoughts and unnecessary stress that eats them from inside. This does not only have emotional consequences, but also physical in terms of increased pain.

A rheumatologist and assistant professor at the University of Texas's Southwestern Medical School in Dallas, Scott Zashin, says:

*"We are so used to multitasking that we find it difficult to sit down and turn off our thoughts."* He adds, *"Meditation is not a quick fix; it takes time."*

You may be wondering how meditation can help relieve your pseudogout pain. A study was conducted and published in the October 2007 issue of *Arthritis Care and Research*, in which individuals with rheumatoid arthritis meditated for 45 minutes every day for six consecutive days a week. This practice continued for a period of 6 months. The results were surprisingly in their favor; it was found that their psychological stress reduced by almost 30 percent.

While there are some types of meditation that involve deep thought, chanting, and breathing exercise, you certainly do not have to spend a lot of time to see the results. As a matter of fact, those who have not tried meditation generally think of it as being something quite complex. Contrary to this belief, meditating is actually very easy. Spending just a few minutes each day contemplating in a quiet environment can help you release your stress, cope better with pseudogout, and develop an overall positive attitude to life.

Here are a few tips for those people who may be interested in starting meditation:

*Educate Yourself* – The best way to start is by educating yourself about all the available meditation options. You can begin by reading books, researching online, and by getting in touch with a meditation expert. This way, you will be able to learn about how people with pseudogout or other arthritic conditions deal with pain through meditation.

*Get an Instructor* – If you are new to meditation, consider enrolling yourself into meditation classes, as this is easiest way to learn how to meditate. You will also be able to ask any questions you may have and get answers from professional therapists.

*Focus On A Single Thing* – Repeating a certain word or counting your breaths is an effective way to prevent your mind from wandering away. Professional therapists recommend choosing a single word that makes you feel relaxed and calm, and then repeating that word to ensure that you are properly focused throughout your meditation session.

*Forget the Time* – Does meditating for 15 minutes seem impossible to you? Quit keeping track of time. Instead, try to focus on the breathing or that particular word and sit quietly. This way, you will be able to extend the duration of your meditation sessions.

*Forgive Yourself* – It doesn't matter if you have to focus on something else when you should be clearing your mind. When thoughts come, acknowledge them and then try to redirect your focus. After all, meditation is about doing the very best of what you can. It is referred to as a practice for a reason; the more you practice, the better you will become.

*Know Your Limits* – Meditation is not a treatment; rather, it's a way to cope with your condition as effectively as possible. Understand that the pain may not go away with meditation, but you will grasp the skills needed for you to better manage it.

*Get Meditation to Work* – You do not need to meditate for hours and hours to see the positive results. In fact, on very busy days, you may not have the time to settle down for lengthy sessions of meditation. There is nothing to worry about; all you have to do is sit down for five or ten minutes in a quiet place where you can concentrate on your breathing. This alone can give you a much-needed boost.

For the best results, follow a healthy diet and get involved in regular physical activities.

***Remain Committed*** – There is no point of meditating unless you are committed to your meditation practice. Don't forget that you are trying to make your life better, and not trying to perfect everything. Aim low, and take one step forward at a time.

***Get Help*** – When starting meditation for the very first time, people typically need some kind of formal instruction. You can get formal instruction by visiting a therapist who leads a meditation group. You can also refer to books if you are the type who prefers to learn on your own. There are also numerous digital media available, which you can watch and follow course. Regardless of which method you choose, you need to start from the very basics to ensure that you learn effective techniques and methods to meditate properly. There is, however, one major advantage of joining meditation groups. You will most likely meet people who have pseudogout and are trying to meditate to gain control over their condition; this way, you will be able to share ideas with them on how they cope with the pain on a daily basis or when having flares.

## Pseudogout and Meditation

You may be wondering; how can something as straightforward as taking just a few minutes breath, think, and focus on your psychological and physical state bring relief to your painful joints?

Surprisingly enough, an increasing number of experts are now hopping onto the meditation bandwagon and recommending this ancient practice as something that can really help in battling chronic pain.

Also referred to as mindfulness therapy, it consists of numerous variations based on the basic meditation concept. Some of these variations have been practiced and are being studied for effectively managing arthritis pain, according to Andrea Minick Rudolph, who is a meditation expert as well as a therapist in Harrisburg. Rudolph is also an experienced deep muscle massage therapist and a Zen Buddhist priest. She practices daily meditation while training others to utilize the techniques in order to effectively manage their arthritis pain.

*"We don't choose to have arthritis, but we can choose how to respond to it and to cope with it,"* states Rudolph. *"By not allowing pain to define our lives, we can change how we view and relate to pain. That's mindfulness – we are changing our feelings and thoughts around pain."*

### What is Meditation?
As an umbrella term, meditation is used to refer to a number of mind-body practices to relieve anxiety, stress, pain, or insomnia. According to a 2007 National Institutes of Health survey, as many as 20 million Americans now frequently practice some type of meditation.

*"It's important to note that arthritis pain will always be there. With mindfulness/meditation, as with any alternative therapy, it's the perception of pain and the management of pain that makes the difference,"* says Rudolph. *"The ability to deal with thoughts around pain is the important step to reduce and manage pain."*

Mindfulness and meditation methods and practices can be carried out on your own or as a part of a group led by a professional therapist. These techniques include:

- Deep-breathing exercises to increase relaxation
- Cognitive-behavioral therapy (discussing your emotional issues with a therapist) to encourage positive thoughts
- Focusing on your body's sensations or body scanning
- Yoga-based meditation

- Use of mantras or chanting or use of mantras (repeating phrases or words)
- Guided imagery or concentration on positive visual images or scenes
- Contemplative walking, common in Buddhist traditions and in Japan

### How Does Meditation Work?

Steven Rosenzweig, an emergency medicine doctor who also very keenly studies the benefits associated with meditation explains how meditation really affects pain as well as other arthritis symptoms:

*"One, it's possible for the pain intensity in these patients to be lowered. Two, the cycles of pain escalation can be moderated. And three, the pain may be there, but it becomes less intrusive on one's life or thoughts."*

Through meditation therapy, individuals with arthritis can gain the ability to manage their pain and gain an understanding that they can use to experience life to its fullest despite the pain.

*"We learn how to stay connected with what is pleasant and nourishing in life. We call these the interstices – the places in between the painful moment"*, says Dr. Rosenzweig *"Our experience becomes enriched and enlivened by moments of enjoyment and pleasure."*

That fits together with a unique type of meditation Rudolph uses along with many other therapists. She calls this technique 'open awareness'. The goal here is to not suppress any thoughts about the pain, but focus on trying and *"letting them in and observing them."*

The ultimate goal of meditation is to relax the body and the mind while engaging in feelings about not only the pain that you experience, but also other challenges that you may be facing. This experience will help you to release tension that is trapped inside you and tap into the unlimited reserves of positivity – despite suffering from a chronic illness such as pseudogout. It is important to understand that when you focus too much on negativity, particularly on the feelings of loss of well being and health, it only worsens the pain. Regarding this, Rudolph says,

*"Meditation helps bring things into present-moment awareness, to see where we are, and assess things in that moment."*

Rudolph explains that it is very easy for a person with pseudogout to fall victim to the negative feelings associated with pain. There are many professionals out there who are trying to bring meditation techniques to more and more people with pseudogout and other types of arthritis.

*"My job is to bring them out of a victim mentality and bring them to a place where they feel they have a choice. With our thoughts, we create a reality. We can actually change our neural pathways by changing the way we think,"* explains Rudolph.

## A Scientific Approach to Meditation

A lot of people within the medical community concur with Rudolph's opinion that meditation practice can indeed help individuals with arthritis and can empower them to take full control over their pain and emotions. We aren't just talking about opinions here. As a matter of fact, there are scientific studies that reveal the positive results of implementing meditation practice for individuals with pseudogout/arthritis pain.

The number of people who are skeptic about meditation is decreasing slowly as more and more positive results of meditation are surfacing. In fact, a therapy called mindfulness-based stress reduction (MBSR) has been showing promising results in arthritis patients. This therapy has been created by Dr. Jon Kabat-Zinn at University of Massachusetts Medical School's Center for Mindfulness.

Meditation enables people who are struggling with chronic pain and the psychological effects caused by it (anxiety and depression, for instance), to identify the positive features of their life.

*"This particular program [MBSR] is a health intervention. Not to turn people into talented meditators, but to teach people to improve their moment-to-moment experience in life. You have pain, and then there's the reaction to that pain. Often, that reaction can make the pain worse."*

Mindfulness-based stress reduction therapy (MBSR) can disrupt the vicious cycle, says Dr. Kabat-Zinn.

*"You bring in some choices and practices that help to tone down the pain experience. With pain, tension can begin to arise in points of the body even distant from the point where the pain is originating. So we can attend to the body, make adjustments and relax certain areas before escalation to a crisis point."*

## Research Validates Meditation

Dr. Rosenzweig, working with his colleagues, has published numerous research studies after studying the benefits of MBSR for arthritis patients and those people who suffer from chronic pain as well as pain associated with flare-ups. He published a study back in 2010 in the renowned Journal of Psychosomatic Research. This study comprised of 100 or more patients who were using meditation to gain better control over their pain management. All of the patients who participated in meditation sessions saw quantifiable enhancement in their quality of life as well as a reduction in psychological distress. This contributed to a reduction in the intensity of pain and their functional limitations. Results did vary slightly among the participants; however, Dr. Rosenzweig is certain that the therapy can indeed be useful in treating arthritis pain.

He says, "Understandably, we have thoughts around pain; catastrophic thinking. The response of the body is to become tenser. So mindfulness practice allows us to step back from negative thinking. We just come back to the present time, become calmer, and respond by working with the current situation."

On the other hand, there are other studies that have indicated that mindfulness-based practices not only play a part in helping people to focus more on positive thoughts while boosting their mood; but they also tend to enhance physical symptoms. For instance, a study in 1998 was led by Dr. Kabat-Zinn, who assisted psoriasis patients undergo phototherapy alongside meditation. People who didn't use medication saw lesser improvements compared to those who did.

Recently, another study was published by a distinct group of researchers at the Massachusetts General Hospital who used magnetic resonance imaging (MRI) to fully document the effect of an 8-week MBSR course.

The area of participants that underwent MRI included those regions of the brain that were responsible for learning, memory, self-referential processing, emotion regulation, and perspective. The images of these areas actually became denser after a 2-month practice of meditation.

## Meditation Can Reach Where Medication Cannot

Even though there are some really powerful medications available, affected individuals still tend to struggle with inflammation and pain, both psychologically and physically. Meditation also assists people with arthritis manage their symptoms more effectively. Alex Zautra, a professor at Arizona State University in Tempe, has a PhD in clinical psychology. He says:

*"The problems of these patients go beyond what can be done with medicines we now have to treat them. Pain is not only a physical experience but an emotional one. Learning to manage those emotions is important for people with inflammatory disorders."*

It is not clear as to how and why meditation has positive effects on a person's neurological system; however, evidence such as brain scans further acknowledge the medical community's belief on the advantages offered by meditation. *"We are more certain than ever that this is for real,"* says Zautra.

79

Zautra started to study meditation as a type of complementary therapy for people with arthritis after discussing this with a rheumatologist. He studied over 144 patients who had RA and divided the individuals into three, random groups. One group received guidance on healthy living, while the second group received information on utilizing standard cognitive-behavioral therapy to better manage their pain, whereas the third group was directed towards mindfulness/meditation practice.

Patients who were in the cognitive-behavioral therapy group were found to show the greatest improvement in their self-reported measurements of pain. There was also a reduction in their IL-6 levels. IL-6 is an inflammatory cytokine that is involved in immune system response.

The meditation group showed the highest increase in their ability to manage the pain effectively, leading Zautra to the conclusion that such practices do in fact help people deal with pain and live a much more normal life.

## The Benefits of Meditation

*"[Meditation] allows a person to become aware of and come to terms with all of their feelings. It helps you see and feel all of your emotions, not just the painful ones. In our study, we gently urged our patients to begin to open their minds to positive emotions, not just negative ones."* says Zautra.

Regardless of whether practicing formal or informal meditation, a person who suffers from arthritis-type conditions such as pseudogout, rheumatoid arthritis, or other similar chronic pain conditions can build a positive outlook towards life and manage their pain with dignity.

The benefits of meditation come with persistent meditation. While it will not replace your regular medications, physical activity or a healthy diet, meditation can and will have a powerful effect on these treatments and your overall quality of life.

*"Dealing with the whole person is essential to healing,"* Zautra says. *"The most compassionate we can be with ourselves is to accept a situation, manage it, and not let it define you as a person."*

# Chapter 6: Staying Active

It doesn't matter if you suffer from a certain form of arthritis such as pseudogout; you can still become an avid exerciser and give up being a couch potato – while it will take a lot of courage and effort from your side, it will be totally worth it.

According to a study from the University of North Carolina in 2008, individuals with arthritis who exercised for around an hour twice a week experienced reduced pain and enhanced their mobility significantly compared to those who were not involved in any physical activity whatsoever. Not only this, but the Canadian Medical Association Journal stated that exercise greatly reduces numerous health issues, including the possibility of cancer, heart disease, diabetes, obesity, osteoporosis, and depression.

Do not let inertia, inexperience, or any arthritis-type condition prevent you from exercising.

Vonda Wright, an orthopedic surgery professor at the University of Pittsburgh Center, says:

*"Contrary to popular belief, there is never an age, skill level or stage of arthritis so bad that you can't do something constructive for your mobility."*

The chairperson of the physical therapy department at the Seton Hall University in NJ agrees with Vonda Wright:

*"Most people with arthritis don't exercise because they're in pain – not realizing that exercise is a powerful and effective pain reliever. It eases inflammation, improves energy and promotes the flow of feel-good, pain-relieving chemicals like endorphins."*

There is no reason why you should be delaying starting your exercise program. This chapter will help you to understand how you can prepare and stick to an effective exercise regime to reduce your pain and enhance your joint performance.

## Getting Ready

Before you put on your sneakers and head out, it is important to follow the steps given below to ensure that you start off safely.

***Consult Your Doctor*** – It is crucial that you consult your rheumatologist as well as the general physician about your plans to start an exercise program. They may advise you against some types of activities based on your medical history. Cedric Bryant, the chief science officer at the American Council on Exercise, says:

*"Ask your doctor for specific suggestions, including how long and hard you should exercise," says Bryant. "If they are unable to do so, seek the help of a physical therapist or certified professional trainer who has extensive experience working with people with arthritis."*

***Establish Modest Goals*** - While it is great to have big dreams, such as aiming to lose a hundred pounds or so, it is important to establish practically achievable goals. If you don't set smaller goals, you may become discouraged and quit all your efforts altogether.

***Understand What You Should Wear*** – One of the most important thing that you need is a pair of extremely comfortable shoes. They should fit you perfectly – visit a walking or running store and get yourself the ideal pair. A good pair of running or walking shoes will ensure that your particular needs are met for the majority of aerobic & strength-training workouts. While it is fine and you can walk in a running shoe, avoid running in walking shoes. When shopping for shoes, wear the socks that you will be wearing during your workouts, and try the shoes for a minimum of 10 minutes or so.

Loose-fitting clothes such as cotton shorts, t-shirts, sweatshirts and sweatpants are OK to start with. However, if you believe that you'll be sweating a lot or would be working on your gym equipment, it is best to go for perspiration-wicking, form fitting attire to avoid getting your clothes caught up in the moving parts.

If you are going to be using a bike, use a helmet along with gel-padded gloves as well as a comfortable seat to avoid any injury.

## Taking a Step Forward

Now that you are ready to take the big step and start exercising, it is important to establish a clear plan that you can follow. Here are a few strategies that can help you unleash your inner exercise enthusiast:

***Work with an exercise buddy*** - Ask a friend, a relative, or a colleague to join you on your exercise program. Exercise becomes more enjoyable and less burdensome when someone accompanies you. An exercise partner will also help you to remain committed to your goals.

***Reward Yourself*** - Research clearly shows that whenever a person is rewarded for his or her "good behavior", including in the case of exercise, he or she will feel much better about it and will be in a position to repeat it.

*"Instead of rewarding yourself with food, do something that builds on your new healthy habits. For example, book a massage or a pedicure, [or go] window shopping at the mall with a friend,"* says Doreen Stiskal.

***Commit To Your Cause*** - Make your physical activity a part of your day that is non-negotiable.

*"Schedule it in your calendar as you would a doctor's appointment, and do everything you can to stick to your plan,"* says Haveren, a sports psychologist based in Atlanta. *"It's all too easy to fall off the fitness wagon when you start skipping workouts. I recommend trying to exercise for at least 10 minutes, even on bad days."*

**Pick the Ideal time** - According to Bryant,

*"You'll enjoy your workout more if you don't do it when your symptoms are at their worst. For example, if you're most stiff when you wake up, then exercise after work. Or if you're exhausted at the end of the day, work out in the morning."*

## Time to Start!

There are numerous types of exercises that are principally effective for people with arthritis, including pseudogout. The following five exercises can be great for you:

**Walking** – Walking is an exercise that is safe for almost everyone, including those individuals who suffer from severe forms of arthritis. Also, the only equipment that you will need for this exercise is a pair of comfortable shoes; not only that, there is no training required at all!

**Water workouts** - Those people who are heavier can benefit greatly by swimming or indulging in water aerobics. The great thing about water workouts is that it reduces the stress on your joints as you workout. Thus, if you feel a lot of pain when walking, such as when going through pseudogout flare up, consider opting for water activities. If you have access to a heated pool, this would be even better as warm water works wonderfully in reducing joint pain.

**Stationary/Recumbent Cycling** - Both stationary and recumbent bikes enable you to increase your heart rate while putting little pressure on the knee joints and the hip. If your balance is dicey, the safest option for you is to choose a recumbent bike. Similarly, if you are new to exercise, overweight, or are exercising following a knee surgery, the latter option remains ideal. An upright bike is great as it lets you spin faster, meanwhile, it is usually the best for an exerciser who is injury-free and experienced.

**Yoga and Tai Chi** – Yoga and Tai chi are known to enhance balance and flexibility – these two areas are those with which arthritis patients often struggle to maintain. Both the techniques are also very gentle on the joints. Why not check with your local fitness or community centers to see if they host yoga and tai chi classes? If you prefer to be alone, you may want to exercise by watching a Yoga or Tai Chi video tutorial.

***Resistance Training*** - Resistance training is a must for people who have pseudogout or other forms of arthritis. Contrary to common belief, weights are indeed an excellent option, as Stiskal explains:

*"The key to using them safely is to have proper form and to lift the correct amount of weight for your strength level. If you're not sure, ask a physical therapist or personal trainer to teach you. Strong muscles absorb the shock that would otherwise affect your joints. It's like the difference between walking barefoot on a cold floor and wearing warm, padded slippers."*

Some of the good ways to build lean muscle is by using rubber resistance bands and strengthening equipment at the gym.

## Don't Give Up

Your motivation may start to fade after a few months, while your joints may become extra achy. It may be that your schedule gets out of your hand. Nonetheless, you have to ensure that these issues do not break your momentum. Here are a few tips how you can continue sticking to your plan despite the following excuses that you may come up with.

**"The joints hurt."** Various studies have shown that exercise does reduce the symptoms of arthritis, including pain and stiffness. According to the chief of sports medicine at Los Angeles County University and Southern California Medical Center, Dr. Vangsness:

*"Exercising releases pain-relieving chemicals, lubricates joints and strengthens muscles that cushion the joints. There's truth to the saying 'use it or lose it.' If you remain inactive, your condition will get worse."*

**"I'm busy."** That's short for saying "my well being and health is not the top priority for me". Spending only a 30 minutes or so every day is an investment that will pay off by protecting you from severe illnesses and will keep your condition from worsening. If you are seriously running short of time, even then it's important to set aside at least 10 minutes at the very least for physical activities.

**"I get bored."** If your physical activity starts to feel like a burden, you need to switch a few things. The best way is to add variety to your exercise program.

## Psyching Up For Exercise

Have you been interested in initiating an exercise program for quite some time now, but cannot get yourself to get into action? This is where the state of mind comes in; the emotional conditioning of a person is as crucial as his or her physical conditioning. Apart from professional athletes, only a few people focus on the mental aspects of their physical fitness regime. Regardless of whether it has to do with overcoming anxiety caused by injury or is just about getting motivated to get fit, changing your mindset can make a huge difference in how you lead your life. With that said, you need to nourish your mind before you can get into physical activity of any kind.

According to a recent study, fear of pain was found to be the causal factor in preventing arthritis patients from exercising; other mental barriers include a lack of enjoyment in exercise as well as a lack of motivation.

*"Participants who exercised and those who didn't both reported arthritis-related pain,"* states the author of the study, Sara Wilcox, a PhD and the associate professor at the department of exercise science at the University of South Carolina in Columbia.

*"Those who were active focused on how exercise increased their quality of life, while those who didn't exercise often had trouble getting past fear and other emotions."* She adds.

87

So how is it that you can get your mind ready and all psyched up for exercise? Here are four tips to help you condition your mind:

**Be Flexible** - Those individuals who were found to have adjusted their physical activity routine in order to accommodate their pseudogout condition had a greater chance of continuing exercise as compared to those who did not.

*"Eschew an all-or-nothing mentality,"* states Judy Van Raalte, a professor of sports psychology at the Springfield College, Massachusetts.

*"If your knees hurt, resolve to walk more slowly. If you're stiff in the morning, then exercise in the evenings. Or cut the length of your workout in half, if you're really sore. Having a Plan B keeps you from giving up when things seem tough."*

**Aim for the Benefits** – During Wilcox's study, those individuals who exercised frequently did so due to the fact that it made them feel good, encouraged weight loss, and made them more capable to move.

*"Reminding yourself of how good exercise is for your health can motivate you to make the effort, even when you're feeling tired, sore or nervous,"* adds Wilcox.

**Soothe Yourself** - Being afraid or anxious can intensify pain; this is why it's crucial to calm yourself before moving on, says Van Raalte.

*"Before you start exercising, spend several minutes breathing deeply while picturing yourself doing your chosen activity,"*

She also recommends getting involved in positive self-talk prior to, and during, exercise; thinking or saying out aloud phrases such as "I can achieve this," and "I do feel the pain, but I have to carry on as this will reduce the pain."

## Four Major Benefits of Exercise

The benefits associated with exercise are much greater than just letting your calories burn after that recent indulgence that you couldn't resist. As a matter of fact, there are numerous reasons why you should be exercising, including the fact that exercise can bring down inflammation due to pseudogout, and other related conditions. It can also significantly decrease the risk of developing other chronic diseases while reducing joint pain.

Here is an overview of four studies that will shed some light on reasons why you should be exercising:

***Exercise Will Keep You Young*** - Even though researchers are not fully clear as to what causes aging, it is a known fact that inflammation has a role to play in the ageing process. A study comprising of healthy men – who were aged between 65 and 74 – was carried out and the results clearly showed that being physically fit and active would reduce the amount of inflammatory chemicals inside your cells. According to researchers at Ball State University's Human Performance Laboratory in Muncie, exercise can control inflammatory chemicals; therefore it may help to bring down the decline in the functioning capability of the human body as a result of aging.

***Exercise Enhances Endurance & Heart Health*** - Arthritis and its numerous forms, such as pseudogout, fall into the category of inflammatory conditions. This inflammation is linked to an increase in the risk of developing heart disease, while this inflammation also has an effect on the joints. It also affects arteries too, thereby causing an increase in blood pressure. Exercise can get the blood flowing and can increase not only your endurance, but also can enhance your overall cardiac health. You can enjoy a lot of benefits of exercise without practicing high-intensity aerobics. Researchers at the University of Pennsylvania learned that getting the blood flow to increase sufficiently kindles an anti-inflammatory response within the blood vessels' cells, assisting them to keep the arteries open.

***Beneficial for Arthritis & Diabetes*** - The same type of inflammatory chemicals that are associated with rheumatoid arthritis (RA) can block the insulin receptors, rendering the cells resistant to the benefits of insulin. Insulin resistance can lead to diabetes. According to a latest study, exercise tends to decrease the level of inflammatory chemicals while increasing the quantity of insulin and glucose used by the body rather than stored by it, by almost 16 percent. By reducing inflammation, you can alleviate joint pain as well as reduce the risk of developing diabetes.

***Every Bit of Exercise, Not Calories, Counts*** – While reducing your calories does help in losing weight to some extent, it does however slow down the metabolism. Combining a calorie reduction plan along with increasing your physical activity level is undoubtedly a smart way to shed weight. A lot of people try to cut the intake of their calories; however, a study comprising obese postmenopausal women at Wake Forest University revealed that focusing on diet alone for a period of 6 months did bring down the total amount of fat in the abdominal area; however, it did reduce the amount of inflammatory compounds in a way that exercise does. To reduce inflammation and boost your metabolism, you need to follow a two-branched approach comprising of both.

## Warming Up For Exercise: Stretching

Stretching is a great way to warm up prior to exercising and it is a practice that you would have learned in your grade school's gym class. Today, healthcare professionals debate on the efficiency of stretching. While some research shows that stretching does improve flexibility, there are some that indicate that stretching to warm up may actually obstruct athletic efficiency, reduce muscle strength, and in many cases, increase the chances of injury.

The facts? Stretching is useful, says Amy Ashmore, who is a training physiologist with American Council on Exercise. Stretching benefits individuals with arthritis by lubricating their joints and enhancing them in addition to maintaining their range-of-motion.

*"Static stretching (stretch and hold) works best after a five to 10 minute warm-up or after you exercise,"* states Ashmore.

A warmed up muscle is capable of stretching longer and can endure additional stresses imposed upon it, states Duane Knudson, a professor and chair at the department of health, physical education & recreation at the Texas State University.

*"Stretching at the end of the cool-down phase, after exercise, also helps to maintain long-term flexibility benefits,"* he adds.

## A Whole New Method of Stretching
Replacing the static stretching techniques with the dynamic stretching methods prior to exercise increases the results and helps you warm-up better. Also referred to as "sports-specific" stretches, the dynamic stretches imitate movements utilized in certain sport or a physical activity. Dynamic warm-ups prepare your body for physical activity by increasing the blood flow and muscle heat range.

If you're planning to play tennis, for instance, you'll need to practice side as well as front lunges during your warm-up activities – these are the actions that you'll be using to reach for the tennis ball.

If you want to go for a walk, you'll want to begin with a gradual pace and pick up speed gradually.

*"Light, gentle, rhythmic movements work best for the average person,"* explains Ashmore. *"Go through a shallow range of motion (i.e. a half-squat vs. a full squat) until you're thoroughly warmed up."*

Nevertheless, you should always talk to your doctor or consult your physical therapist before trying new techniques of stretching.

## Exercise: A Great Medicine

Exercise used to be considered as something slightly more than sport. But in the past several decades, experts and enthusiasts alike have come to realize that exercise isn't just intended for fun; in reality, it has numerous benefits for the body and mind, too.

As a matter of fact, studies have revealed that exercise can be highly effective, or in certain cases, more effective than the medication used to prevent diabetes, heal depression, and reduce cognitive decline. Sometimes, maintaining or losing weight only requires bringing about some changes to the lifestyle, such as implementing an exercise regime; this is particularly important when medications alone don't do the job.

Today, as science is constantly discovering many ways in which exercise improves health – right down to a cellular level – there's only a little doubt that working out (exercising) can be downright therapeutic.

That's not to imply that any single style of working out will cure all illnesses. While performing some exercise is better than performing none at all, *"certain types are especially well suited for certain health goals,"* explains Pete McCall, an exercise physiologist at the American Council in Exercise (ACE).

*"Choosing the right activity – as well as the correct duration, intensity and frequency – can help you achieve the best results, and allow you to make the most of your time."*

Read on to find out the best kind of exercises for specific health goals.

### *Your Goal: Increase Energy*
The Type of Exercise – If your goal is to increase your energy levels, perform almost any exercise you wish as long as it's easy on your joints. Researchers at the University of Georgia reviewed more than 70 studies that spanned 50 years and found that people who carried out strength training, aerobics, or mobility exercises

for no less than 10 minutes daily saw a significant improvement in their energy levels after a period of 4 to 8 weeks.

Frequency: Four or more days every week

Intensity: Mild

How this works: Exercising stimulates the cardiovascular and nervous systems while boosting your brain's production of neurotransmitters that make you feel good. Michelle Olson, a professor of exercise physiology at Auburn University's Human Performance Research laboratory in Montgomery, Ala, explains:

*"Physical activity targets the basis of exhaustion through reducing the extent of – and in most cases even solving – energy-sapping illnesses including obesity, substantial blood pressure, arthritis and depression, "* claims Olson.

Researchers at the University of Georgia tested the theory that exercise can treat fatigue in thirty-six adults who had persistent fatigue; these individuals were not regular exercisers. They split the participants into three groups. One group was involved in 20 minutes of moderate-intensity cycling by using an exercise bike 3 times a week for a period of six weeks. The second group followed a similar routine, but at a simpler, low-intensity pace. The third group didn't exercise at all. Both the teams that exercised reported a 20 % increase in their stamina by the end of this study. The study was published in a journal called Psychotherapy and Psychosomatics.

### *Your Goal: Reduce Pseudogout/Arthritis Pain*
The Type of Exercise: Exercises that involve gentle stretching, such as yoga and Tai Chi, are excellent options. In addition, water-based exercises such as water aerobics or swimming are ideal exercise options when you are experiencing a flare. Combine this with strength to gain longer-term rewards.

Frequency: If possible, carry out these exercises for at least thirty minutes a day and 3 times a week; but doing so for just twenty minutes, 3 times a week can also be quite beneficial.

Intensity: Mild

How this works: The last thing you should be doing during a flare is ceasing all physical movements, while it can be quite tempting to do so in order to feel less pain.

*"When an individual exercises, the body releases pain-relieving substances, including endorphins,"* says McCall. Even though this mechanism is not properly understood, physical activity does appear to bring down cellular inflammation, which could further worsen inflammatory conditions, such as arthritis.

Evidence: A report inside Cochrane Database of Systematic Reviews viewed 32 studies comprising of people with osteoarthritis (OA). It was found that land-based exercise was as effective for knee pain as the effects of non-steroidal anti-inflammatory drugs (NSAIDs), such as ibuprofen or naproxen. Another report on eight trials that studied exercise's effects on OA, published in Data Based Medicine, found that physical exercise did actually reduce the pain people felt by as much as 50 percent.

### *Your Goal: Reduce Pain and Fatigue Associated with Fibromyalgia*
The Type of Exercise: A mixture of aerobics, lifting weights, and flexibility training is undoubtedly highly effective.

Frequency: Start off with the maximum duration that you can achieve, even if it is five minutes each day.

Intensity: Mild

How this works: Fibromyalgia is just starting to be understood by the healthcare community, and as a result of that, experts aren't totally sure how physical exercise alleviates fibromyalgia-related pain.

However, the applicable theory is that during exercise, your body releases endorphins (chemicals that are considered to be natural pain relievers) states Jacob Teitelbaum, the medical director of nationwide Fibromyalgia and Fatigue Centers. Exercising also increases vitality by stimulating cardio and central nervous systems.

Evidence: The evidence of this is so far limited; however, it is growing rapidly. The results of the study comprising of twenty women with fibromyalgia were published inside Archives of Physical Medicine and Rehabilitation found that when strength training and aerobics were combined, it resulted in improvements of the symptoms, especially a reduction of fatigue.

*Your Goal: Relieve Depression*
Type of Exercise: Aerobic exercises such as walking, biking, jogging, aerobics, and swimming.

Frequency: A minimum of thirty minutes, 3 times every week. The effects of aerobic exercises heavily rely on the amount of time that you spend exercising. The more you exercise, the better the results will be.

Intensity: Moderate to Strong.

How this Works: *"There's good evidence that aerobic activity increases the brain's levels of serotonin, dopamine and norepinephrine -- three neurotransmitters that elevate mood,"* explains Stacey Rosenfeld, who is a licensed clinical psychologist and runs a private clinic, while she is also a staff psychologist at the Columbia University Medical Center in NYC. She adds:

*"Completing even a short workout gives you a sense of accomplishment, and self-esteem is tied to a reduced incidence of depression."*

Several studies have been carried out in the benefits of exercise in reducing depression, which often haunts people with pseudogout and other arthritis-related illnesses. The findings have revealed that exercise does have a positive impact on a person's mental health. A study was carried out at Louisiana State University's Pennington Biomedical Research Laboratory in Baton Rouge. This study found that women who lead sedentary lifestyles initially and began exercising - moderately - reported an enhancement in the quality of their life. The quality of life is an accurate measure of a person's physical and mental skills that are needed to cope with the challenges of everyday life. The more the women exercised, the greater they felt, even if they did not shed weight.

### Your Goal: Maintaining/Losing Weight
Type of Exercise: Aerobic exercises such as walking, biking, jogging, aerobics, and swimming.

Frequency: A study conducted at Duke University revealed that moderate exercise performed for just thirty minutes a day is enough to prevent a person from gaining weight. Nonetheless, numerous other studies have figured out that the majority of people who want to lose weight successfully exercise for 60 minutes or more of cardiovascular exercises, such as walking no less than 5 days per week.

Intensity: Mild or moderate.

How this works: In order to maintain weight, the concept remains the same as the one involved when losing weight: you have to burn more calories than the amount of calories you take in.

*"Study after study shows that most weight-loss winners keep their calories in check through consistent, steady aerobic exercise – and the majority of the time, the activity of choice is walking,"* explains Olson.

However, she notes that those people who add resistance training to their exercise regime do a great favor to themselves. This is because the muscle they gain speeds up their calorie burning process, thereby making it much easier for them to lose or maintain weight.

As many as 90 percent of all participants in the National Weight Control Registry – which is a group of more than three thousand people who have managed to successfully maintain a 30-pound weight loss for a duration of 1 year (minimum) – consider their exercise programs to be crucial to their weight management efforts. According to them, burning 2687 calories per week is equal to walking 4 miles every day.

### Your Goal: Reduce Bone Loss/Prevent Osteoporosis
Type of Exercise: Any type of weight-bearing exercise that requires your bones to support your entire body's weight. Resistance training is also extremely effective; however, many types of aerobic exercises, such as walking, also work fine.

Frequency: At the bare minimum, you need to carry out resistance training for 15 minutes, 2 to 3 times per week.

Intensity: Mild or Moderate.

How this works: *"Weight-bearing exercise puts stress on your bones. Your bones' cells react by creating additional bone mass,"* says Michael Gloth, who teaches at the John Hopkins University School of Medicine as an associate professor of medicine. He is also known for helping to develop the National Osteoporosis Foundation's guidelines for osteoporosis patients. Dr. Gloth states that those people who already suffer from arthritis-type conditions should supplement their workout sessions with calcium and vitamin D supplements. Alternatively, they can also turn towards dietary forms to ensure that their body prevents further loss of bone, thus effectively rebuilding the bone density.

German researchers conducted a long-term study and found that a diverse exercise program comprised of jumping, running, stretching, and weight-training 4 times a the week can be extremely helpful for individuals with pseudogout, arthritis in general, and osteoporosis. This was proven by the results of 86 premenopausal women who were a part of the study. These women had osteopenia; however, the diverse exercise program helped to preserve their bone density over a period of two years, as compared to the group who was not as active.

The group of women who performed no exercise lost as much as 2.3 percent of their bone density, the group which exercised frequently saw no reduction in the density of bone. This study was published in Archives of Internal Medicine.

## Guidelines for the Intensity of Exercise
In order to determine the intensity of your workouts, please adhere to the following guidelines.

*Mild*: After mild exercise, you should be capable enough to have a thorough conversation with a person. If you use a heart rate monitor, aim for around 40 to 50 percent of the maximum heart rate.

*Moderate*: After moderate exercise, you should be able to say short sentences (such as 'I am fine '), however, you may find it difficult to establish a detailed conversation. For those using a heart rate monitor, aim for no more than 50 to 70 percent of the maximum heart rate.

*Vigorous*: In vigorous exercise, you are normally on the edge of your comfort zone; you would find holding a conversation difficult. When walking, your pace would be 4 miles an hour or more. For those using a heart rate monitor, aim for no more than 70 to 80 percent of the maximum heart rate.

**It is crucial that you get in touch with your physician before you start off with any type of exercise program.**

## How to Make Exercise a Regular Habit
There are three ways in which you can make your life better – by decreasing stress, sleeping better, and reducing pain–and surprisingly enough, exercise can help you to achieve all three.

Once you are prepared to perk up the quality of your life and develop exercise plans, you would surely want to create a daily physical exercise routine before you actually exercise. How can you make that? Always remember that a lifestyle that involves regular exercise is lived one step at a time; the quality of life that you wish to enhance would depend on each of these steps.

Know this: Your feelings and thoughts support you what you do (actions). Your actions, on the other hand, help you take those steps we talked about above. Once you start to take the steps again and again, this behavior translates into your habit. Read on to find out how every little step that you take adds up to make a complete lifestyle.

Learn to become conscious of your emotions, particularly the ones that you relate to your experience of exercise. Tune into them and try to comprehend the joy and well-being benefits of being active. It is much easier to be active you're your mind enjoys the results of the exercise.

Imagine walking just around the block to fetch your mail and visualize playing with your own kids or grandkids. Let these thoughts stir creativity, so that you start to develop numerous other feel-good exercise routines.

Learn to live in the moment. The present is the only place where you can genuinely be active. Events take place in the present not in the time that has passed or the time that is to come in the future. When you learn to utilize the opportunities present right in front of you, such as walking up a ramp at a mall even when an escalator is present, or riding a bike when you can drive. All of these opportunities present ways for you to get fit and develop a healthy lifestyle. When you start taking care of each of these little things, you will automatically be setting yourself up for success with bigger goals, such as your daily exercise routine.

## The Ideal Time to Exercise

Some people prefer to start their day only after they exercise, while there are some who prefer to head out for a walk right after dinner. How would you know which time is ideal for exercise? Is one more effective than the other?

One thing that is the most important in determining the ideal time for you to exercise is when you feel at your best. Not only will you get the most out of your exercise – both in mental and physical terms – but you will also be able to adjust your schedule accordingly to implement your daily exercise routine.

Achy and stiff joints tend to slow people with arthritis in the morning. Thus, if you wish to exercise first thing in the morning, you should give yourself some time after you wake up and take a warm shower to help your joints become supple.

If you prefer to exercise in the evening, then carry out a few experiments where you determine how your body responds. If your pain gets worse during the day after you increase your physical activity, the following fatigue can wear you down more. If you find that you are exhausted or if you feel as if your joints are sore, leave exercise for the next day. Don't forget to pick a better time though. However, do try to get at least a little exercise every day.

If a pseudogout flare appears for a couple of days, ask your physician or therapist on how you should modify your exercise routine.

*"Even when symptoms are at their worst, you don't need to stop exercising,"* explains Vonda Wright, who works as an orthopedic surgeon at the University of Pittsburgh Medical Center's Center for Sports Medicine. She adds, *"Maybe it's not the right time to go for a brisk walk, but you could try using a recumbent bike. I also recommend doing water aerobics in a warm pool – it will feel soothing and will keep you moving."*

## The Benefits of Walking
What is there about walking that isn't likeable? It is easy, it's good for your joints – and best of all, and it's completely free! In addition, the fact that it is good for your overall physical and

mental health cannot be denied. It is a type of aerobics and a study conducted at University of Tennessee revealed that those women walked regularly had lesser body fat as compared to those who did not.

Walking also considerably reduces risk of blood clotting. This is because the calf tends to act like a pump, pumping blood from the feet and the legs back to the heart, thereby causing a reduction on the load exerted on the heart. There are numerous other benefits of walking.

For instance, walking greatly improves the circulation of blood throughout the body. It prevents the development of numerous heart diseases, increases the heart rate, reduces blood pressure and fortifies the heart.

Numerous studies were conducted at the at the University of Colorado and the University of Tennessee that revealed that post-menopausal women that walked around 1 to 2 miles each day successfully brought down their blood pressure by as much as 11 points with a time period of 24 weeks. Those women who walked for 30 minutes every day eliminated the risk of a stroke by 20 percent, and by as much as 40 percent after having increased the duration.

Walking also decreases the risk of suffering from fractures. At Brigham and Women's Hospital in Boston, a study consisting of post-menopausal women revealed that half an hour of walking every day reduced the risk of hip fracture by almost 40 percent.

Walking also enhances life span. According to a latest research from the Medical School at University of Michigan and the Veterans Administration Ann Arbor Healthcare System, those people who exercise regularly in their 50s and 60s have a 35 percent less chance of dying over the next decade, as compared to their non-exercising counterparts. This percentage increases to 45 percent for those who suffer from certain chronic health conditions.

Walking supports the joints. It effectively tones the muscles, which then support your joints, particularly the abdominal and leg muscles. Even the muscles of your arm will be toned if you pump them when walking. Walking stops the bone mass loss, especially for those people who have osteoporosis. Michael Schwartz of Plancher Orthopedics & Sports Medicine in New York, explains:

*"One of the well-known orthopedic phrases is 'life is lotion and lotion is life.' Walking starts that 'lotion' moving through the joints."*

Most of the cartilage in joints does not have a direct supply of blood. These joint cartilages get their nutrition from joint fluid (synovial), which circulates when we move. The impact that results due to compression or movement compression, such as when walking, tends to 'squish' the cartilage, thus bringing nutrients and oxygen into these areas. If you do not walk, the joints get deprived of this essential fluid that will speed up the deterioration process.

Walking enhances the flexibility and strength of the muscles, thereby increasing their range of motion, and transferring the pressure as well as the weight from your joints to your muscles. The muscles are supposed to handle some of the weight – and can reduce arthritis-related pain.

Excess body weight exerts extra pressure on the joints. If you start walking on daily basis, not only will you strengthen your muscles – making them capable of carrying your additional weight, but you will also be reducing the unwanted weight – a two-in-one advantage.

# Chapter 7: Everyday Solutions

Those individuals who are suffering from arthritis and other related conditions, such as pseudogout, can and do experience significant problems when performing day-to-day tasks. In certain cases, when there is a lot of inflammation and pain, such as during a flare, simple activities such as cleaning the house and doing other chores around the house can become quite difficult.

This chapter will reveal valuable information that can help pseudogout patients to lead normal lives and perform tasks in a way that is smart and efficient.

## Smart Methods To Use When Working Around The House

To reduce the trauma induced on your joints and the body in general when cleaning your house, it is important to warm up first by initially walking around your house. After you have warmed up your body, follow the guidelines given below to simplify the cleaning process.

### *Safe Way to Bend*

Most Common Mistake - Bending from your waist

Bending is often required when performing the following tasks:

- Unloading the washer, dishwasher and the dryer
- Collecting and picking up items
- Washing the dishes
- Ironing
- Cleaning below the furniture
- Scrubbing tubs
- Making beds

Safer solutions:

- Try to get in the habit of bending your knees and not the back. Slightly flex your knees and keep a slight hollow in the back
- When you are standing up, you can reduce the back pressure by placing one foot on a slightly elevated surface; for instance, on a step stool
- When unloading things, use a technique called the 'golfer's lift' - All you have to do is to kick back the leg that is opposite to your extended arm
- Kneel or ask for assistance from others if you have to do tasks down at the floor-level

### Reach Out Correctly
Most Common Mistake - Reaching out with an arm fully extended (stretched).

This is often required when performing the following tasks:

- Cleaning the walls or windows
- Dusting
- Picking objects from the floor
- Reaching for overhead shelves
- Washing the dishes

Safer solutions:

- Keep your arms closer to the body in order to reduce the strain on your shoulders
- Bring objects to your waist's level as an alternative to reaching out with your arms
- Utilize poles and wands that have extended handles when dusting
- Avoid excessive arm and back extension by utilizing a strong stepstool when trying to reach for overhead items

### Kneeling Properly
Most Common Mistake - Kneeling down on both knees.

Some of the tasks that require a person to kneel down on both of their knees:

- Washing floors
- Cleaning low cabinets
- Scrubbing showers and tubs

Safe solutions:

- Kneel on a single knee and keep switching knees regularly to reduce and disperse the pressure
- Wear kneepads if possible or cushion your knees with soft pieces of clothing

### *Lift Lightly*
Most Common Mistake - Lifting a lot of weight, or having poor posture when lifting.

Some of the tasks below require a person to lift:

- Hoisting laundry baskets
- Lifting the cleaning buckets or boxes
- Moving the furniture
- Taking the trash out

Safe solutions:

- Before you lift something, squat beside it and while keeping your back straight, rise up straight, slowly and steadily
- Hold an object closer to your body in order to reduce the strain on your back
- Whenever possible, use carts (wheeled) to move around heavy things
- Do not lift any heavy or awkwardly-shaped loads alone; find someone to help you.

*Pushing Painlessly*

Most Common Mistakes - Pulling objects instead of pushing them; leaning with your waist; over-extending your arms; bending the wrists.

Some of the common tasks where you have to be cautious in order to avoid the above-mentioned mistakes are as follows:

- Mopping
- Sweeping
- Vacuuming
- Moving objects

Safe solutions:

- Instead of pulling objects, push them
- Keep your head up and correctly in line with the spine
- Always avoid thrusting the arm back and forth. Alternatively, try to walk with a broom or a mop or even a vacuum with your arms in a relaxed position.
- When sweeping, make use of a flat-headed broom and make sure you push with its leading edge. Sweep all the areas into a single pile and then pick it up using a long-handled dustpan or a vacuum cleaner
- When mopping the floor, alternate between the mopping styles to vary the stress on your muscles. For instance, switch between rocking side-to-side and figure 8s.
- Avoid imposing stress on your wrists by ensuring that they are kept straight, and not bent when holding the handles.

## Fighting Germs – Common Myths

A lot of drugs that control inflammatory types of arthritis, such as pseudogout, do their work by repressing an immune system that is overactive, which is the reason behind the attacks on joints and the associated damage. For those who are taking these medicines, there are both advantages and disadvantages.

Firstly, these types of medications relieve inflammation and reduce pain while curbing the progression of the disease; however, they also make a person more susceptible to numerous infections from bacteria, germs, and viruses.

If you are consuming these medicines, you need to make sure that you are taking the right steps to protect yourself from germs. It is especially important to take prudent measures when you are likely to come into contact with pathogens, which are likely to make you ill.

Read on to find out what works and what does not work when it comes to protecting yourself from the germs and viruses.

*Myth Number 1* – A kitchen sponge can be sterilized by heating it up in a microwave.

This does not work if you are depending on the radiation let out by the microwave alone. Philip Tierno, who is the director of microbiology and immunology at New York University's Langone Medical Center and is also the author of a book called The Secret Life of Germs: What They Are, Why We Need Them, and How We Can Protect Ourselves Against Them, explains that microwaves are untrustworthy germ killers due to the fact that these appliances have certain dead spots where the radiation is not capable of reaching. Even when a turntable is being used, it is quite possible that the bacteria and the viruses will remain on the kitchen sponge. Do not forget that a kitchen sponge is among one of the most germ-infested surfaces in the entire household.

However, Tierno also states that there are many other reliable ways to properly sterilize the kitchen sponge in a microwave:

Begin by immersing the kitchen sponge in a dish of water that is microwave-safe. Put this dish in the microwave and turn it on for 4 minutes on a high setting. The microwave will then heat the water to around 150 degrees Fahrenheit, a temperature that is sufficient to kill many germs and bacteria. However, it is crucial that you allow the sponge to cool down before you pick it up.

On the other hand, you could also soak the kitchen sponge in a solution containing two and a half tablespoon of bleach mixed with 4 glasses of water.

***Myth Number 2*** – It is acceptable to wipe the counters with a sterilized kitchen sponge.

If you use a dish sponge to wipe your counters, it is very likely that your kitchen only appears to be clean, says Elizabeth Scott, a microbiologist who serves as a co-director of the *Center for Hygiene and Health in the Home and the Community* at Simmons College.

*"In reality, what you've done (and I've tested this), is you end up spreading bacteria around your kitchen,"* she says, while recommending that you use the sponge only for dishes and encourages us of paper towels for wiping the counter.

***Myth Number 3*** - Antimicrobial agents in cleaners and soaps are ineffective in killing germs and that they can make your immune system weaker and the germs stronger.

The idea that a person can clean themselves sick is known as hygiene hypothesis. Even though there is some evidence that indicates that the malfunctioning immune system, such as due to asthma, allergies, or eczema, can increase as a result of us not being exposed to all kinds of germs during childhood; some experts still consider this idea as being flawed.

*"My informed feeling based on the work that I've looked at is that [the rise in some diseases is] not because we're too clean,"* says Elizabeth Scott. *"If you take it to its logical conclusion, if being too clean is compromising our health, let's look at a community in Zimbabwe and look at what's happening there. That's a community that's definitely not able to be too clean, they're experiencing a huge onslaught of microbial pathogens all the time, and they're very, very sick."*

While such kinds of theories are useful during research, when it comes to everyday life, *"Certainly, if you're already immune-compromised,"* says Scott, *"you cannot be too clean."*

It is generally not necessary to use cleaners that contain germicidal ingredients on floors and windows, as these things are relatively free of viruses and bacteria. However, if you have an infant who starts crawling, that is when you also need to clean the floor. If you have a pet and it has defecated or vomited on the floor, then it becomes an absolute must to clean up that area using disinfectants.

***Myth Number 4*** - You are more likely to get a cold from a person who sneezes only 2 feet away in the office or on a plane.

That is very much possible, agrees Scott, but it is not too likely. Based on a number of studies she carried out to determine how people contract germs, a person is more likely to fall ill after coming into contact with a virus, and then touching their face several times a day. *"We, all of us, touch our faces so many times a day that we inoculate our eyes, in particular, and then the virus moves down into the nose,"* says Scott.

The tear ducts in the eyes are extremely vulnerable, as they do not possess the defense systems against germs that are present in the mouth or the nose. Therefore, if a person touches something contaminated and then rubs their eyes, they are most susceptible to get infected.

## Coping with Arthritis

## Building Resilience in Life
Diana Reyers is a mother of two who has some experience of bouncing back from a downward spiral caused by the diagnosis of rheumatoid arthritis (RA) back in 2005. After being diagnosed with this type of arthritis, she could not continue working her management job. Thus, she resumed education in an attempt to find a less demanding and less stressful career. She even opened

up her own spa in the year 2008; however, that too had to go when she developed osteoarthritis in both her thumbs.

*"I was left with little money and an immense feeling of being unfulfilled,"* Reyers recalls.

In 2010, when she was having a really bad neck spasm, she explains, *"I lay down to rest and had an epiphany: I was not going to beat arthritis, but I could live with it in a better way."*

She started to work with a rheumatologist to come up with effective ways and medication and this made her take a U-turn on the way she was leading her life. She became a professional life coach and is now extremely happy with her rewarding career that spares her plenty of time for herself and the family.

So what is it that makes people like Diana Reyers make the most of their lives despite having a painful disease such as pseudogout or other forms of arthritis? It is resilience.

According to Robert Wicks, a psychologist Robert Wicks, 'Resilience is the ability to learn from and rebound from challenges, adversity and stress.'

When a person becomes resilient, they gain the ability to keep themselves going despite their mental or physical state, the pain, and the grief. It allows them to develop coping mechanisms such as acceptance, optimism, and faith that they can set things right and lead lives comfortably and happily without a hint of frustration.

Building resilience is even more important for people who have arthritis, explains Robert Wicks, who is a professor at the Loyola College in Maryland and the author of the book Bounce: Living the Resilient Life.

*"Chronic disease poses regular, and often immense, psychological and physical setbacks,"* he adds. "You have to be able to cope with them in order to care for yourself. Resilience is

the difference between making arthritis one part of your story and [allowing it to be] your entire narrative."

### *Remedy for Alleviating Pain*

Various researches show that those individuals who have greater resilience also have faster recovery rates. These people are also efficient at managing pain, and are less vulnerable to chronic anxiety and depression. Not only this, but they also have an overall advantage when it comes to good health as compared to those people who have lesser levels of resilience. For instance, once study published in the renowned Journal of Consulting and Clinical Psychology observed 300 women with arthritis and figured out that women who answered higher on resilience questionnaires experienced less pain as compared to the ones that scored low.

Yet another study that looked at 275 patients was published in a journal called Annals of Behavioral Medicine. These patients suffered from osteoarthritis and among them those who had the greatest number of characters related to resilience were the ones most probable to show self-worth; for instance, they were the ones most likely to see a physician on a regular basis while exercising regularly. Lesser pain and an enhanced ability to carry out everyday tasks was the benefit enjoyed by resilient individuals.

*"Resilience impacts thoughts and, therefore, behavior in profound ways. A less resilient person experiencing a flare might think, 'well, I can't exercise,' or 'my doctor isn't helping me enough.' A resilient individual thinks, 'How can I improve my situation? What can I do to get moving again?'"* explains Dr. Elizabeth Lombardo, a physical therapist and a psychologist based in Chicago.

A certain set of 'coping skills' are needed to implement resilience in a person's personality. These skills also help by reducing stress levels and the hormones that further aggravate pain resulting from pseudogout pain.

### Building Your Resilience

The majority of experts agree on the statement that some people are naturally resilient; however, various researches show that resilience can be developed to boost buoyancy. *"It's a skill that can be developed and honed over time,"* explains Wicks.

If you are willing to build your resilience, you can try the following strategies and bounce back stronger and better.

Focus on the positive side - studies reveal that optimism plays an important role in building resilience. The more hopeful a person feels, the more resilient they will be. In order to boost optimism, follow the guidance of Dr. David Hellerstein – a professor of clinical psychiatry at the College of Physicians and Surgeons in NYC, when he says, *"Reframe your experience so that you're aware of the negative, but focused on the positive."*

He advises people to ask themselves the following three questions: *"Does this provide new opportunities? Can I look at this differently? Is there any good to come out of it?"*

Learn from your experience - if you suffer from a chronic disease, you are probably more resilient already than you think yourself to be. Patricia O'Gorman, a psychologist in New York, specializing in resilience and trauma, says *"When you're dealing with a new setback, that's the time to ask yourself, 'How have I dealt with problems in the past? What worked, and which strategies should I skip this time?'"*

When Lisa Emrich, a pianist, developed arthritis, she followed the approach of O'Gorman, learning from her experience with sclerosis.

*"I saw a doctor right away, kept getting tested until I had a diagnosis, and worked with my physician to formulate a plan – in this case, medication plus occupational therapy, which ultimately allowed me to return to playing the piano,"* she explains.

Increase your knowledge – in order to become resilient, you need to get as much knowledge as you can about your health condition. Ask a lot of questions when visiting your physician or rheumatologist. In addition, it is recommended that you read material containing information on pseudogout and arthritis.

*"Learning boosts resilience," says Hellerstein, "The more you learn about how best to live with your condition, the more control you have. Control as well as resourcefulness gives you the confidence to move forward in the face of adversity."*

Find your bliss – Get some time off and do the things that make you happy. Just like resilience researchers from the University of California have said, *"emotions like joy, satisfaction and interest ... provide individuals with a sort of 'psychological time-out' in the face of stress and help them perceive the 'big picture' of their situations."*

Exercise – exercise does not only have physical benefits, but also mental. It greatly decreases depression, enhances sleep and augments the level of mood-improving chemicals, such as that of brain-derived neurotrophic factor (BDNF). BDNF is a protein that is known to improve health of the brain. Studies have also revealed that people who are physically fit do not have intense spikes in their blood pressure when they are exposed to stress and stress hormone cortisol.

Get support – There are certain support systems that can play an important role in developing resilience.

*"If you don't feel like you have to go it alone, it's much easier to push forward when the going gets tough," says Wicks.*

If you are not in the habit of asking for assistance, you need to understand that asking for support does not indicate that you are weak. It is very likely that your loved ones and friends are waiting for you to ask them for support.

Count your blessings – at the University of California, researchers reviewed as many as 225 studies and they found that people who expressed gratitude or maintained a journal in which they wrote down the things that they were grateful for actually felt more optimistic, autonomous, and connected. Wick says,

*"Gratitude makes you think about what you have, which, in turn, keeps you from focusing on what you don't have. When you feel blessed, it's easier to keep going – no matter what you're up against."*

## Managing Stress

Chuck Currie knows a lot about stress management. Currie has worked with homeless people for over 17 years, doing a wide variety of tasks ranging from serving sandwiches to running the entire operations at a family shelter based in Portland, Oregon. He has seen people suffering from numerous disabling health conditions and has even witnessed teenagers die from AIDS.

Around two years back, Currie shifted to St. Louis and altered his career path, starting a Masters of Divinity program. He started to experience a surge in his stress levels. Besides that, help did not come as easily.

*"Moving, changing careers and entering seminary were all stressful things that happened in quick succession,"* Currie explains.

Coincidently, Currie also began to experience pain and swelling in his hands, feet, and knee joints. In some cases, his symptoms aggravated so much that it became difficult for him to get out of the bed. Twice, he had to rush to the emergency room as a result of his flares. Chuck Currie has psoriasis; he had also developed psoriatic arthritis – a joint condition that occurs in around 23 percent of people who have psoriasis.

Based on Currie's experience, stress can be extremely difficult to manage, especially for people who have autoimmune diseases.

This is because most biological pathways that light up the stress response consist of the same pathways that are involved in the malfunctioning of the immune system.

For those people who have arthritis or other types of inflammatory conditions, stress causes certain chemicals to be released in the brain as well as the body, thereby triggering flares, pain, and more inflammation. To make things worse, a few of these chemicals, such as cortisol, elevate the danger of developing numerous types of chronic conditions, including obesity, heart disease, depression and anxiety, which tend to further increase stress.

After entering this cycle, it becomes extremely difficult to manage your health – akin to jumping from a helium balloon that just keeps rising out of reach. Fortunately, whatever goes up may be brought down, and the same is true for stress.

Stress can be reduced through numerous techniques, and the system's natural balance and overall health can be restored to its former glory.

### *Blame the Chemical Messengers*
What is stress? Stress is defined as our response to a particular stressor or demand, explains Hans Selye, a MD, commonly known as the 'Father of Stress'. Long waits at a post office, traffic jams, and conflict with family members all account for stress. Most people tend to be affected by such stressors every day.

For those who have arthritis, they would know that chronic health conditions such as this could result in more stressors piling up. For instance, stiff joints slow down a person in the morning, causing him or her to be late for work. A favorite activity such as needlepoint can become aggravating. The joint pain can also cause you to stay awake all night, hence making you cranky and sluggish the next day. All of these things lead to stress overload.

When everything is smooth in life and there are no hurdles, the body's organs along with the chemicals that they develop are totally balanced. However, when the body is subjected to a stressor, for instance, if your car skids a little on a slick road, the body responds by making some chemical messengers active, explains George Chrousos – the chief of the National Institute of Child Health and Human Development, at the Pediatric and Reproductive Endocrinology Branch of National Institutes of Health.

It all begins in hypothalamus – the main gland in the brain. The hypothalamus excretes a hormone that reaches the pituitary gland, causing it to release another hormone, which in turn signals our adrenal glands to let go of stress hormones, such as cortisol, epinephrine, and norepinephrine.

All the processes takes place within a few seconds, and are the reason behind our fight or flight response. As long as these chemical messages are working normally, they help the body and mind deal with all kinds of problems throughout our lives.

Nevertheless, if any of these messengers fail to do their job correctly, the balance is disturbed. Stress hormones have a part to play in controlling other types of chemical messengers that are known to influence biological processes, including body temperature, blood pressure, heart rate, metabolism, appetite, mood, fertility, sleep, pain perception, and the responses of the immune system.

In the case of Chuck Currie, his problem of psoriasis was a result of excessive stress. As a matter of fact, a Finnish study has found that men, especially, were more prone to experience psoriasis and joint pain when under stress.

*"It's cyclical,"* states Currie, *"because the stress level will impact my arthritis, and the arthritis will impact my stress level."*

### Pathways Transport Stress
Due to the fact that people who have arthritis have already experiencing many inner body stressors (which affects production

of cortisol), researchers want to examine how the levels of cortisol are affected by the external stressors – both in people who have arthritis as well as those who do not.

At the Milton S. Hershey Medical Center at Pennsylvania State University in Hershey, researchers studied how a particular stressor, such as loss of sleep (6 hours instead of 8) affected 25 young and healthy students. After a week with less hours of sleep, the blood test of the students revealed decreased levels of cortisol and an increase in the cytokines. Cytokines are chemicals that cause inflammation. Such changes are also found in people who have rheumatoid arthritis even if they have sufficient hours of sleep.

Even though experts believe that a lot of factors, including heredity, are likely to contribute to an individual's development of conditions such as arthritis, stress is considered to be a prime suspect and reason behind it. Why?

The immune response and the stress response share a few pathways.

*"The processes that fire up the immune system and lead to the proliferation of inflammation-inducing chemicals are the same processes that are stimulated by stress,"* states Alex Zautra, a PhD and an Arthritis Foundation-funded researcher as well as professor at Arizona State University.

Some experts even believe that the chicken-and-egg predicament is involved. For example, hiccups in the immune system can lead to stress. On the other hand, stress itself can lead to immune system hiccups in those people who are vulnerable. Now the question is: Who's vulnerable? According to experts, this depends on way individuals are 'wired'.

## Some People Have Been Wired for Stress
There are various theories that have been coined by researchers explaining how people tend to become wired, or more

117

appropriately 'miswired', for stress. For example, prolonged exposure to chronic stressors such as having to live with arthritis or looking after aging parents seems to have an impact on chemical messengers.

Researchers at Ohio State University measured a particular inflammatory chemical in adults and discovered that those people who were looking after their chronically ill spouse were four times more likely to have the inflammatory chemical in their blood as compared to those who were not in such a situation. The elevated inflammation marker continued to remain in their systems even years after their spouse had died, thereby indicating that the stress circuitry changes tend to have long-lasting effects.

## Trauma Can Result in Delayed Stress

Physical or even psychological trauma, such as losing a loved one or going through sexual abuse, for instance, can also alter the stress circuitry in a number of people. According to some researchers, post-traumatic stress disorder (PTSD) takes place when through the initial trauma, norepinephrine is released which mark the memories strongly or too deeply in the brain. People who have PTSD have flashbacks of memories of the trauma they suffered in the form of nightmares. They also develop insomnia, which tends to keep the norepinephrine and stress levels high for a long period since they experienced the trauma. As many as 56 percent of people with fibromylagia who have some symptoms of PTSD have been found to have a high level of stress and pain as compared to those who have no symptoms of PTSD.

## Hormones Have a Huge Impact on Women's Stress

Research confirms that women are more vulnerable to stress than the opposite sex, with the estrogen hormone being the culprit. While it is true that immense stress can suppress the production level of this hormone (this is among one of the reasons why female athletes tend to stop menstruating when they train intensively), it has been found that estrogen affects the brain and makes it more sensitive to stress. However, men with rheumatoid arthritis have increased pro-inflammatory estrogens and a decreased level of the male hormone testosterone (an anti-inflammatory hormone), in comparison to men who do not have rheumatoid arthritis.

## Socio-Economic Status Can Be an Important Factor

It has been found that people who have low education levels suffer from an increased number of acute and/or severe daily stressors. This has been found by a latest study from Wake Forest University School of Medicine in North Carolina. For example, rain can be an inconvenience at most to someone who works in an office; however, it means lost wages for someone who works outdoors (such as a laborer). Also, the socio-economic status tends to determine the resources that a person has when dealing with stress, states the leader of the study Dr. Joseph G. Grzywacz. Mental health counseling, massages, and health-club memberships are not exactly easily accessible for those who are struggling to make ends meet.

*"Stress is really a component of every disease,"* explains James Rosenbaum, the professor of inflammation research at Oregon Health & Science University and the chair of the Division of Arthritis and Rheumatic Diseases.

Here are a few adverse effects as a result of stress:

*Increased abdominal fat leading to obesity* - Researchers have now found that excessive levels of cortisol steers fat towards an individual's middle. This is the place where fat is deposited and where it builds up near the abdominal region. Even in fairly thin, healthy people, chronic stress can cause some fat to build up in the middle areas.

Excessive abdominal fat and obesity in general are major risk factors for diabetes and heart disease, and this form of fat emits profuse amounts of pro-inflammatory chemicals, which increase inflammation.

*Diabetes* – The leading cause of diabetes is obesity. However, chemical imbalances that result from stress, whether a person is obese or not, may trigger the development of diabetes type 2. Scientists at the University of Washington in Seattle have found that an increase in fear, a lack of control and depression can elevate levels of insulin and glucose, both of which are dangerous for diabetes.

***Cardiovascular Diseases*** - Acute stress and anxiety increase blood pressure and restrict blood vessels, both of which are major cardiovascular concerns. Stress is also known to increase levels of triglycerides, cholesterol, and homocysteine – all of which indicate some kind of heart disease.

***Sleep Disturbances & Insomnia*** - A nationwide sleep poll was conducted in 2003 and as many as 72 percent of individuals with arthritis reported problems sleeping. These problems included the loss of deep, recuperative sleep that can be credited to higher stress levels. The increase in stress levels can also cause insomnia. People can then get further stressed about their lack of sleep, thereby putting them in yet another cycle. In turn, Sleep deprivation can avert the brain from correctly modulating pain.

***Mental Health Challenges*** - Stress modifies neurotransmitters that regulate emotion and mood, leaving an individual more vulnerable to anxiety and depression. Depression also deteriorates inflammatory conditions, such as pseudogout. People who were depressed were found to experience twice the amount of pain as compared to those who were not depressed, according to a study conducted by researchers at Stanford University Medical Center, California.

*"Depression itself has been associated with elevations in proinflammatory cytokines,"* explains Zautra. *"That's independent of whether the person has arthritis. So when you combine these factors, they become a more potent brew."*

## Managing Stress
There are numerous stress reduction methods that can be practiced in an attempt to decrease the damaging effects of stress.

The aim is to come up with strategies and methods that work well in reducing your stress levels. There is no single strategy for reducing stress that works well for everyone. One thing that works reasonably well for your friend may not work for you.

Nonetheless, it is crucial to know that you have the resources available to deal with the disease (pseudogout) and by feeling empowered, you will be able to have a greater semblance of control.

Boost your techniques of managing stress by following the tips given below:

### *Let Go Of Self-Defeating Thoughts*
Giving judgments about your body and health can cause you to develop a stress response. Saying things such as 'I'm too young to experience pain" or that "I should have been stronger than this," will only make things worse.

MBSR or Mindfulness-Based Stress Reduction can help people to let go of such feelings. The process requires you to understand and recognize stressors, and will enable you to let them float away, explains Trish Magyari, program director of MBSR at University of Maryland Medical Center's at the Center for Integrative Medicine in Baltimore.

*"People learn that self-defeating thoughts are doorways to the pit of their own personal despair. If they can learn to see the doorway, they can learn that they don't have to go through it,"* states Magyari.

### *Focus and Breathe*
One popular MBSR technique used to manage stress is known as diaphragmatic breathing. This is done by taking deep breaths consciously – inhaling through the nose, and exhaling out from the mouth, allowing the diaphragm to expand.

### Skeletal Muscle Relaxation

This progressive muscle relaxation technique involves holding, tightening and then releasing various muscle groups from the face to the toes, while the attention should be focused onto a certain phrase, image, or word in order to relax during breathing.

### Vent Out

Stress can also be released by letting go of anger or any negative emotions that may have collected inside you. A study was carried out to determine the effects of maintaining a journal by renowned researchers at the Southern Methodist University in Dallas. They discovered that those people who spent at least 20 minutes every week for a period of four weeks brought down their blood pressure levels significantly, thereby easing the physical reaction they had as a result of stress. By writing down things that trouble you, or by calling up a friend and discussing it with them every now and then, you can vent out negativity and prevent it from building up inside you.

### Limit Your Sweet Intake

When a body is subjected to stress, it craves carbohydrates as a result of the extra production of hormone cortisol. While it is true that carbohydrates and sweets discharge endorphins that make you feel good, these effects tend to be short-lived. As the body starts to crave more sweets, the person is put in the habit of consuming carbohydrates and sweets and therefore ends up in a difficult-to-break cycle.

Researchers at UCSF studied several women who had cortisol in high levels and discovered that these participants craved sweets, and ended up eating large quantities of them after a particular stressful event. To lower cortisol levels, incorporate fresh fruits and vegetables into your diet along with proteins.

### Switch Off the TV and Exercise

A Sedentary lifestyle and behaviors, such as watching too much television, is linked with weight gain as well as an elevated risk of developing other health conditions, including the onset of stress.

A recent study conducted at the Harvard University in Cambridge revealed that those men that watched a lot of TV, greater than 40 hours each week, were at a three times greater risk of diabetes, as compared to those men who watched it only for an hour every week.

Add variety to your routine and get a break by walking briskly as soon as you feel stress starting to build up. Tai chi and yoga are excellent forms of meditative exercise. Not only are these exercises easy on the joints, but they also provide flexibility and strength while decreasing stress.

According to a study conducted at Reed College in the city if Portland, 90 minutes of yoga can be highly efficient in reducing cortisol levels; on the other hand, various studies have also revealed that 2 to 3 hours of tai chi every week can improve quality of sleep as well as mental health.

## *Medication*

Inflammatory chemicals are known to ignite pain and swelling, and pharmaceutical companies develop drugs that block or target the culprit chemicals in an attempt to reduce inflammation.

For instance, the following biologic response modifiers (BRMs) are known to block TNF-a – a proinflammatory chemical:

- adalimumab (Humira)
- etanercept (Enbrel)
- infliximab (Remicade)

These BRMs accumulate within the joints of individuals who have some form of arthritis, such as rheumatoid arthritis, and contribute to flare ups and damaged tissues. Healthcare researchers are now reviewing whether stress reduction methods themselves can work similar to a BRM and effectively block the accumulation of proinflammatory cytokines among those people who have autoimmune diseases.

If certain stress-relieving methods, such as breathing techniques or sticking to a healthier diet, do not work, a physician may be able to provide you a short-term relief for your acute stress or severe anxiety condition through medicines.

To keep stress under control, Currie utilized certain meditative prayer practices along with exercises. Now that he has become a parent, he has an additional stressor to cope with.

Together with his wife, he is now experiencing not only twice the stress, but also double the joy after his wife gave birth to twin daughters last year.

Even though not all stress can be avoided, some stress helps you to become a new person altogether – learning and growing. You can, however, you can look for strategies and ways that help you conquer the detrimental stress or the stress overload so you become less vulnerable to any flares.

## Arthritis and Parenting

Parenting is not easy at all, even for those who are completely healthy. Parenting requires you to be present for your kids at all times, day or night.

A painful condition such as pseudogout can hamper your ability and role as a parent. If you have children that require additional attention, and if you have pseudogout, then the following strategies may help you a lot:

### *Remain Involved*

If you have pseudogout, you may not be able to play a one-on-one game with your children; however, it is important to spend quality family time with your kids as it helps you to bond with them. As a parent, develop and involve in activities that both you and your kids can enjoy - without experiencing the pain due to arthritis. Consider playing board games, taking a stroll with them in the park, or going to a movie with them.

### Be Honest About Your Condition
*"Hiding it creates a sense of shame,"* states Mark Lumley, a clinical psychologist as well as a professor of health psychology at the Wayne State University in Detroit. He adds, *"What's more important is to show how you cope with it by reaching out for support and medicating wisely. Kids learn about dealing with illness in a positive way."*

### Remain in charge
Being a good parent does not have anything to do with your physical condition.

*"You can still be a heck of a good parent even if you're struggling with pain,"* Lumley explains. *"Good parents communicate, counsel, teach and discipline their children."*

### Set Priorities in Life
Focus on those things that matter to you. Let go of the rest or delegate it to someone else.

*"Save your energy for what you can do,"* states Ruth Hall, aged 51, an individual with rheumatoid arthritis, fibromyalgia, and osteoarthritis. *"If I had been told to pace myself in the very beginning, life would have been better for all."*

### Stay Positive
Attitude is crucial – or more precisely, the *right* attitude is important when it comes to establishing a strong relationship with your children.

*"If you become defeated by arthritis, your children will feel defeated as well,"* states Annmarie Cano, a clinical psychologist at the Wayne State University.

# Conclusion

Even though pseudogout can be a painful disease, with proper management and care, its symptoms can be kept under control.

The majority of people that develop pseudogout are unaware of how the condition can restrict their day-to-day activities, especially as it continues unchecked. This is exactly why it is imperative that you transform your lifestyle, including the diet and physical exercise routines to ensure that your body remains healthy and fights off any disease.

To accomplish this, proper awareness through education is important. This book has been designed to educate individuals with pseudogout as well as caretakers who look after people with pseudogout.

A very important factor that should be taken into account is that if the individuals with pseudogout are helped by family and friends in dealing with their condition, they would have a better chance of successfully dealing with the pain and inflammation, as well as the stress that follows.

It is a well-known fact that pseudogout flares can be quite painful; a person's ability to function normally may be hampered significantly. Hence, they would require and would certainly appreciate any help they can get from those around them. So if you are a pseudogout-affected individual, do not feel shy in asking for help. Meanwhile, this book includes guidelines, advice, and strategies that can make your life blissful and give you a greater semblance of control over your behavior and life in general.

It is recommended that you refer to this book each time you are feeling down for inspiration and tips. We hope that you will find this book to be of an immense value and we wish you all the best in managing your health condition.

# Published by IMB Publishing 2015

- Turmeric (Recipes?)
- Infrared heating pad
- Game ready ice

pg.17 • GCQ6 supplement

2 serv • Fish / fish oil supp. pg 31
per week

- probiotics - Smoothie (Straw, ban, yogurt, spin, honey)
- massage
- nuts / seeds (Almonds / Pistachios)
- Bell peppers
- olive oil
- Beans
- weight loss
- move at work
- cut caffeine / caffeine free Tea
- WATER
- Vitamins
- Stretching
- Brace
- massage
- warm bath

- exersize - achievable goals
- comf. Shoes

- personal Trainer

- Resistance training

53112951R00072

Made in the USA
Lexington, KY
24 September 2019